MW00510356

THE COMPLETE KETO GUIDE FOR BEGINNERS OVER 50

Everything you need to Live your Ketogenic Diet Lifestyle after 50. Cookbook with Useful Step by Step Easy Recipes with 30-Day Keto Meal Plan for Men and Women to Lose Weight Fast

Jillian Collins

© Copyright 2020 - All rights reserved.

The content contained within this book may not be reproduced, duplicated or transmitted without direct written permission from the author or the publisher Under no circumstances will any blame or legal responsibility be held against the publisher, or author, for any damages, reparation, or monetary loss due to the information contained within this book. Either directly or indirectly.

Legal Notice:

This book is copyright protected. This book is only for personal use. You cannot amend, distribute, sell, use, quote or paraphrase any part, or the content within the book, without the consent of the author or publisher.

Disclaimer Notice:

Please note the information contained within this document is for educational and entertainment purposes only. All effort has been executed to present accurate, up date, and reliable, complete information. No warranties of any kind are declared implied. Readers acknowledge that the author is not engaging in the rendering of legal, financial, medical or professional advice. The content within this book has be derived from various sources. Please consult a licensed professional before attempting any techniques outlined in this book.

By reading this document, the reader agrees that under no circumstances is the author responsible for any losses, direct or indirect, which are incurred as a result the use of information contained within this document, including, but not limited errors, omissions, or inaccuracies.

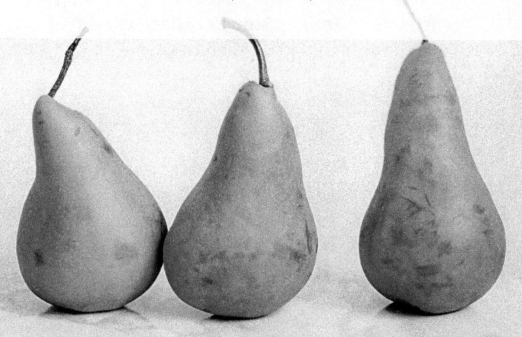

CONTENTS

GRAB YOUR 7 SPECIAL BONUS
IN THE END OF THE BOOK

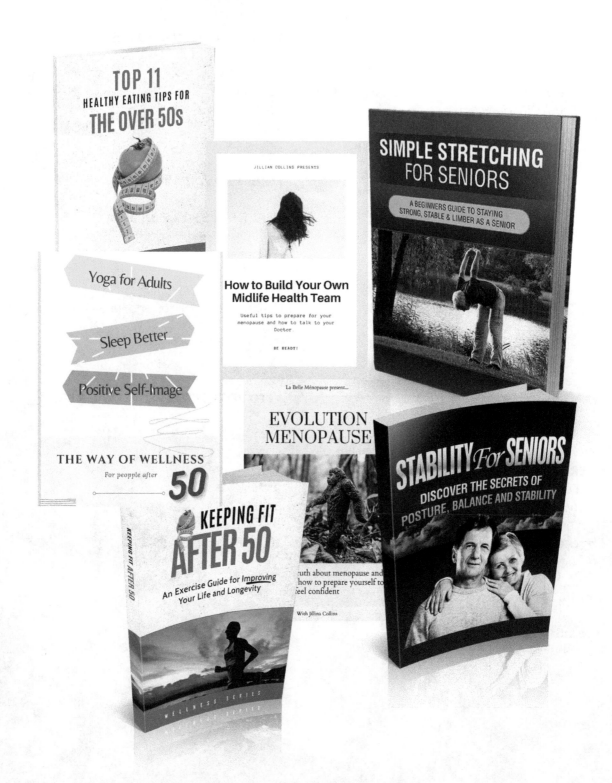

Introduction

Are you over 50 and looking for a weight loss solution that works for you and enables you to eat as much as you desire?

If yes, you are in the right place.

This book was written after numerous consultations with people who reached middle age and began to experience weight gain and other related problems.

I am a Nutritionist with a degree in food science, and I am happy to have been able to help many women and men to achieve their goals. This book is intended to give you a full understanding of how a Ketogenic style can improve your physical and mental state without having to disrupt your habits. You must know that after the age of 50, the body for both women and men begins to undergo various changes, and this is why after the age of 50, a specific diet is necessary. This complete guide has been specifically designed to help men and women over 50 understand why a general ketogenic diet is not adequate but must be adapted and modified.

I am passionate about this way of keeping fit because it is not a classic restrictive diet but allows people to adapt gradually. I live a Ketogenic lifestyle, and although I'm 53 and mother of two boys, I can eat ice cream without feeling guilty and wear the clothes I wore at 30. I also involved my husband, who thought it was not easy, but today he feels invigorated and organizes barbecues with friends every week.

You can achieve this all by a one-of-a-kind diet that can help you burn away excess body fat, take your health and body to a new level, and restore your youth after the age of 50. So why is the Ketogenic diet a miracle for us? Let's start from the beginning. The ketogenic diet is a high-fat, medium protein, and low carb diet. The breakdown of a ketogenic diet is:

Fat: 70 to 90 percent of calories
Protein: 15 to 25 percent of calories
Carbs: 5 to 10 percent of calories

These macro-nutrient compositions make the Keto diet a perfect solution to burn fats in the body. The portion of fats is much more than the standard amount that people are used to consuming. This is where the keto diet gets intimidating as we have been told that fats are bad for health; this is not true. Bad fats are those that are harmful to health, whereas good fats are essential for absorbing vital minerals and nutrients.

Typically, the human body's natural behavior is sugar (glucose), which results from carbohydrate intake through foods. The glucose is then used as fuel by the body to perform its activities. However, glucose is not the most effective and efficient energy source for the body as it brings many serious health issues like coronary diseases, hypertension, diabetes, and obesity (to name a few). Sugar supply doesn't remain consistent in the blood, and that's why we face spikes of energy and become hungry again after eating recently. We also become tired after eating a high-carb meal and often plop down on the couch to take a nap. Glucose from carbs is the first choice of fuel by the body, but when it isn't used and burned through exercises, it is converted into fats, and we gain weight. When our body needs sugar for energy, it doesn't burn the converted in fat, and instead, it sends signals to the brain that provoke us to eat high sugar foods like chips, cookies, etc.

To break the diet routine of consuming more carbs/sugar and become more obese, the body burns off fats through a high-fat keto diet. It means that you are burning fats that have led you to gain weight. The keto diet brings the body into a ketosis state, which is a metabolic state where the body starts processing fats for fuel when carb reserves are depleted. Ketosis transforms fats into ketones that act as a source of energy, and ultimately, as fats keep burning, our weight sheds as well. The change in the body's natural behavior for fuel doesn't let you experience cravings or make you feel hungry, which are annoying side effects of other diets. You will become healthy, fitter, and sharper.

So if you want to know more, keep reading.

THANKS AND WELCOME

What is Keto Diet?

As you'd probably already know, the ketogenic diet is a low-carb diet where you eliminate or minimize carbohydrates' consumption. Proteins and fats replace the extra carbs while you cut back on pastries and sugar.

How Does It Work?

See, when you consume less than 50 grams of carbs per day, your body starts to run out of blood sugar (which is used as fuel to provide your body quick energy). Once there are no sugar reserves left, your body will start to utilize fat and protein for energy. This entire process is known as ketosis, and this is exactly what helps you lose weight.

Compared to other diets, keto has a better chance of helping you lose weight more quickly. The diet is also incredibly popular as you're not encouraged to starve yourself. It would help if you worked towards a more high-fat and protein diet, which isn't as difficult as counting calories.

How the Body Changes When You're Over 50

This isn't going to be fun to read, but once you hit your 50s, you're likely to experience some changes in your body. The most common include:

Weight Gain

According to the Centers for Disease Control and Prevention (CDC), men and women are likely to gain one to two pounds each year as they transition from adulthood to middle age. This doesn't get any better for women as they hit menopause. While the gain in belly fat isn't directly linked to menopause, hormonal changes may cause you to put on a few pounds, depending on the lifestyle and environmental changes.

Metabolism Slows Down

You've probably heard a lot about your metabolism changing as you grow older. That's probably why you can't chow down junk food as you used to when you were in your teens. So, what is metabolism, and how does it affect your body?

In simple terms, metabolism is how quickly your body processes or converts food and liquids into energy. As you grow older, metabolism slows down, and the body starts to convert those extra calories into fat. This is probably why you should skip those convenience meals and start to eat healthier.

Why Should You Switch to Keto?

Once you start to hit 50, you likely don't indulge in strenuous activities anymore, so your body will need fewer calories to function. This is when you should start eliminating added sugars from your diet. Also, most packaged meals or meals provided in the hospital for the elderly are processed and contain empty calories, including mashed potatoes, bread, pasta, and puddings. These foods not only taste bland, but they also lack nutrition to keep your body strong and healthy.

Plus, a low-carb diet that is rich in healthy vegetables and meat will prove to be far better for people suffering from insulin insensitivity and your overall health. Hence, start reading food labels more often and opt for healthier options. A recent study from the Hebrew University of Jerusalem has indicated how eating a diet rich in healthy fats can help you lose weight in the long-term.

Macronutrients and Keto

Macronutrients

The food you consume provides nutrition to the body. Various types of nutrients are present in the food. They are broadly classified into macronutrients and micronutrients. Macronutrients are those nutrients required in significant quantities in the food to provide necessary energy and raw material to build different body parts. These are:

- · Carbohydrates
- · Proteins
- · Fats

Carbohydrates

Carbohydrates are important energy sources of the body. In a Keto diet plan, you have to cut on your carbs to eliminate this energy source and compel your body to spend the already present food stores in your body. These food stores are present as fat in your body. Once your body turns to these fat deposits in the body for energy, you start to lose weight.

Carbohydrates should not constitute more than 5–10% of your daily caloric intake.

Carbohydrates are present in a variety of foods. You should make sure that the small quota of carbohydrates you can consume comes from healthy carbohydrate sources like the low-carb vegetables and fruits, e.g., broccoli, lemon, and tomatoes.

Proteins

Proteins are really important because they provide subunits, which are building blocks of the body. They produce various hormones, muscles, enzymes, and other working machinery of the body. They provide energy to the body as well.

No more than 20–25% of your daily caloric intake should come from proteins. As a rule of thumb, a healthy person should consume about 0.5–0.7 grams of proteins per pound of total body weight.

Many people make a mistake in a keto diet consuming much more protein than they should. This not only puts additional strain on their kidneys but is also very unhealthy for the digestive system.

Eat a good variety of proteins from various sources like tofu, fish, chicken, and other white meat sources, including seeds, nuts, eggs, and dairy (though you shouldn't fill your diet with cheese). Red meat like beef can be enjoyed less frequently. We also suggest you avoid processed meats, which are typically laden with artificial preservatives.

Processed meat refers to meat that's modified through a series of processes, which might include salting, smoking, canning, and, most importantly, treated with preservatives. Such variants typically include sausages, jerky, and salami. As these meats are not even considered healthy for normal diets, we suggest limiting your portions to only once or twice a week.

Fats

In keto, fats serve as the mainstay of your diet. It seems counterintuitive to consume what you want to eliminate from your body, but that is exactly how this strategy works. But before you go about loading your body with all types of fats, keep the following things in your mind:

1. You have to cut on carbs before this high-fat diet can be of any benefit to the body.

1. Fats should take up about 70–75% of your daily caloric intake.

2. Fats are of various types, and you have to be aware of the kind of fats you should consume.

Dietary fats can be divided into two kinds: healthy and harmful. Unsaturated fats belong to the healthier group, whereas saturated and trans-unsaturated fats belong to the unhealthier category. Aside from the differences in their health effects, these fats essentially differ in terms of chemical structure and bonding.

Saturated Fats

Saturated fats drive up cholesterol levels and contain harmful LDL cholesterol that can clog arteries anywhere in the body, especially the heart, and increase the risk of cardiovascular diseases. A diet high in saturated fat has an increased chance of reducing the risks of heart diseases. These fats are mainly contained in animal origin (except fish, which contains a small part). They are also present in plant-based foods, such as coconut oil.

However, coconut oil contains medium-chain fatty acids, which are saturated fats different from animal origin, and therefore considered a healthy food.

- Saturated fats are mostly contained in:
- · Whole milk dairy products, including milk and cheese
- · Butter
- · Skin-on chicken

· Red meat such as pork, lamb, and beef

While there's no doubt that these foods are keto-friendly, they should not be consumed in large quantities, regardless of what diet you follow. It's also worth noting that some saturated fats are rated better in the health department than others. For instance, milk is healthier than consuming red meat. We suggest you limit butter and pork derived from animal fat as they overall tend to be unhealthy.

Unsaturated Fats

These 'good fats' contain healthy cholesterol. Unsaturated fats can most commonly be found in nuts, veggies, and fish. These fats keep your heart healthy and are a good substitution for saturated fats.

Unsaturated fats can be divided into:

Trans Fats: Trans fats, or trans-fatty acids, are a particular form of unsaturated fat. These unhealthy fats are manufactured through a partial hydrogenation food process. Moreover, some studies differentiate the health risks of those obtained industrially or transformed by cooking, from those naturally present in food (for example, vaccenic acid); the latter would be harmless or even beneficial to health.

The industrial foods that contain these hydrogenated fats are mainly: fried foods (especially French fries), margarine, microwave popcorn, brioche, sweet snacks, and pretzels.

While these foods may taste good, they're an unhealthy kind of fat and should be avoided.

Trans fats are known to increase unhealthy cholesterol levels in the blood, thus increasing the risks of cardiovascular disease. The WHO (World Health Organization) has the aim of global elimination of industrially-produced trans fats from food supplies by 2023.

The Main Features of the Ketogenic Diet

Losing Weight

For most people, this is the foremost benefit of switching to keto! Their previous diet method may have stalled for them, or they were noticing weight creeping back on. With keto, studies have shown that people have been able to follow this diet and relay fewer hunger pangs and suppressed appetite while losing weight at the same time! You are minimizing your carbohydrate intake, which means fewer blood sugar spikes. Often, those fluctuations in blood sugar levels make you feel more hungry and prone to snacking in between meals. Instead, by guiding the body towards ketosis, you are eating a more fulfilling diet of fat and protein and harnessing energy from ketone molecules instead of glucose. Studies show that low-carb diets effectively reduce visceral fat (the fat you commonly see around the abdomen that increases as you become obese). This reduces your risk of obesity and improves your health in the long-term.

Reduce the Risk of Type 2 Diabetes

The problem with carbohydrates is how unstable they make blood sugar levels. This can be very dangerous for people who have diabetes or are pre-diabetic because of unstable blood sugar levels or family history. Keto is a great option because of the minimal intake of carbohydrates it requires. Instead, you are harnessing most of your calories from fat or protein, which will not cause blood sugar spikes and, ultimately, pressure the pancreas to secrete insulin. Many studies have found that diabetes patients who followed the keto diet lost more weight and ultimately reduced their fasting glucose levels. This is monumental news for patients who have unstable blood sugar levels or are hoping to avoid or reduce their diabetes medication intake.

Improve Cardiovascular Risk Symptoms to Overall Lower Your Chances of Having Heart Disease

Most people assume that following a keto diet that is so high in fat content has to increase your risk of coronary heart disease or heart attack, but the research proves otherwise!

Research shows that switching to keto can lower your blood pressure, increase your HDL good cholesterol, and reduce your triglyceride fatty acid levels.

That's because the fats you are consuming on keto are healthy and high-quality fats, so they reverse many unhealthy symptoms of heart disease. They boost your "good" HDL cholesterol levels and decrease your "bad" LDL cholesterol levels. It also decreases the level of triglyceride fatty acids in the bloodstream. A high level of these can lead to stroke, heart attack, or premature death. And what are the high levels of fatty acids linked to?

Low Consumption of Carbohydrates

With the keto diet, you are drastically cutting your carbohydrates intake to improve fatty acid levels and improve other risk factors. A 2018 study on the keto diet found that it can improve 22 out of 26 risk factors for cardiovascular heart disease! These factors can be very important to some people, especially those who have a history of heart disease in their family.

Increases the Body's Energy Levels

Let's briefly compare the difference between the glucose molecules synthesized from a high carbohydrate intake versus ketones produced on the keto diet. The liver makes ketones and use fat molecules you already stored. This makes them much more energy-rich and a lasting fuel source compared to glucose, a simple sugar molecule. These ketones can physically and mentally give you a burst of energy, allowing you to have greater focus, clarity, and attention to detail.

Decreases Inflammation in the Body

Inflammation on its own is a natural response by the body's immune system, but when it becomes uncontrollable, it can lead to an array of health problems, some severe, and some minor. The health concerns include acne, autoimmune conditions, arthritis, psoriasis, irritable bowel syndrome, and even acne and eczema. Often, removing sugars and carbohydrates from your diet can help patients of these diseases avoid flare-ups—and the delightful news is keto does just that! A 2008 research study found that keto decreased a blood marker linked to high inflammation in the body by nearly 40%. This is glorious news for people who may suffer from inflammatory disease and want to change their diet to see improvement.

The Calorie and Nutrient Balance

Do you know why else the Ketogenic Diet is good for you, specifically, as someone who just hit 50 years old? You should keep in mind that as a person advances in age, their calorie needs to decrease. For example, instead of 2,000 calories per day, you'll need only 1,800 calories per day. Why is that? Well, when we start to get old, our physical activity significantly decreases. Hence, we don't need as much energy in our system. However, that doesn't mean our nutrient needs also go down. We still need the same amount of vitamins and minerals.

The Ketogenic Diet manages to hit a balance between these two needs. You get high nutrition for every calorie you get—which means that you'll maintain a decent amount of weight without feeling less energetic for day to day activities.

Heart Diseases

Keto diets help women over 50 to shed those extra pounds. Reducing any amount of weight greatly reduces the chances of a heart attack or any other heart complications. Through the carefully selected diet routine, you are not only losing weight and enjoying delicious meals, but you are significantly boosting your heart's health and reviving yourself from the otherwise dull state that you may have been in before.

Diabetes Control

Needless to say, the careful selection of ingredients, when cooked together, provide rich nutrients, free from any processed or harmful contents such as sugar. Add to that the fact that keto automatically controls your insulin levels. The result is a glucose level that is always under control, and continued control would lead to a day where you will say goodbye to the medications you might be taking for diabetes.

How to Start a Keto Diet When You're Over 50?

Once you have decided, the next thing to do is speak to your doctor about it. As discussed, whether or not you're suffering from a medical condition, it's important to speak to your doctor to learn more about the keto diet and if it's right for you. Let's take a look at some steps to take when getting started:

Do Your Research on Keto-friendly Food

First of all, you need to acquire a list of foods to eat and avoid. Depending on your budget and location, some of those foods may be difficult to find. So you may need to look for food alternatives that are also keto-friendly. Moreover, learn how to spot "hidden carbs" in the food items you purchase. Many foods may claim to be keto-friendly but may contain additional carbs or sugars.

Practice Portion Control

Just because you're allowed to eat foods rich in fats and proteins doesn't mean you should eat excessive amounts. Although you don't have to count calories every time you eat, you should practice portion control so you don't go overboard. This is where a high-quality food scale comes in handy.

Be Prepared to Experience Some Side Effects

Although these side effects don't happen to most people, you might be unlucky enough to experience them. One of the most common side effects is a condition known as the "keto flu." You will know that you have this condition if you experience side effects such as headaches, fatigue, irritability, a lack of motivation, brain fog (an inability to focus), sugar cravings, muscle cramps, dizziness, and nausea. However, if you already know what to watch out for, you don't have to worry. Most of these side effects are temporary and will go away. Also, try not to let the side effects discourage you from sticking with the diet.

Exercise

This is optional, but you should take care of your muscles at your age as they start to degrade. You will feel better, your health will improve, and your weight will go down faster.

Consult a Nutrition Specialist

This book is a valuable tool to get an idea of a ketogenic diet, the benefits, and how to avoid classic mistakes. It is a complete guide, with which, if studied well, you will certainly be able to set your diet according to your daily needs. However, consulting a doctor is never a bad idea; you can discuss your opinions and give you valuable advice. I recommend consulting your doctor, especially in health problems and cases where you have never been on a diet.

Tips for Seniors Who Want to Start

Learn How to Count Your Macros

This is especially important at the beginning of your journey. As time goes on, you will learn how to estimate your meals without using a food scale.

Prepare Your Kitchen for Your Keto-friendly Foods

Once you've made a choice, it's time to get rid of all the foods in your kitchen that aren't allowed in the keto diet. To do this, check the nutritional labels of all the food items. Of course, there's no need to throw everything away. You can donate foods you don't need to food kitchens and other institutions that give food to the needy.

Purchase Some Keto Strips for Yourself

These are important so you can check your ketone levels and track your progress. You can purchase keto strips in pharmacies and online. For instance, some of the best keto strips available on Amazon are: Perfect Keto Ketone Test Strips, Smackfat Ketone Strips, and One Earth Ketone Strips.

How to Start a Keto Diet When You're Over 50?

Once you have decided, the next thing to do is speak to your doctor about it. As discussed, whether or not you're suffering from a medical condition, it's important to speak to your doctor to learn more about the keto diet and if it's right for you. Let's take a look at some steps to take when getting started:

Do Your Research on Keto-friendly Food

First of all, you need to acquire a list of foods to eat and avoid. Depending on your budget and location, some of those foods may be difficult to find. So you may need to look for food alternatives that are also keto-friendly. Moreover, learn how to spot "hidden carbs" in the food items you purchase. Many foods may claim to be keto-friendly but may contain additional carbs or sugars.

Practice Portion Control

Just because you're allowed to eat foods rich in fats and proteins doesn't mean you should eat excessive amounts. Although you don't have to count calories every time you eat, you should practice portion control so you don't go overboard. This is where a high-quality food scale comes in handy.

Be Prepared to Experience Some Side Effects

Although these side effects don't happen to most people, you might be unlucky enough to experience them. One of the most common side effects is a condition known as the "keto flu." You will know that you have this condition if you experience side effects such as headaches, fatigue, irritability, a lack of motivation, brain fog (an inability to focus), sugar cravings, muscle cramps, dizziness, and nausea. However, if you already know what to watch out for, you don't have to worry. Most of these side effects are temporary and will go away. Also, try not to let the side effects discourage you from sticking with the diet.

Exercise

This is optional, but you should take care of your muscles at your age as they start to degrade. You will feel better, your health will improve, and your weight will go down faster.

Consult a Nutrition Specialist

This book is a valuable tool to get an idea of a ketogenic diet, the benefits, and how to avoid classic mistakes. It is a complete guide, with which, if studied well, you will certainly be able to set your diet according to your daily needs. However, consulting a doctor is never a bad idea; you can discuss your opinions and give you valuable advice. I recommend consulting your doctor, especially in health problems and cases where you have never been on a diet.

Intermittent Fasting and Keto Diet

What Is Intermittent Fasting?

Intermittent fasting is fasting when you keep away any foodstuff involving calories among ordinary nutritious ingredients. It is not starvation or a way for you to eat junk food with no consequences. There are various methods used to practice IF; they divide time into hours or divide time into days. Since the regiment's response varies from person to person, no process can be called the best.

Knowing that intermittent fasting cannot make you lose the additional pounds you may have instantaneously is essential, but it can prevent unhealthy addictions to meals. It's a nutritional practice that requires you to be determined to follow to get the maximum gain. If you already have a minimum duration to eat due to your schedule, this regiment will suit you like a duck to water, but you will always need to be conscious of what you are eating if you are a foodie. Choose the appropriate regiment after expert guidance. You should see it as a segment of your schedule to get healthy, but not the only component.

Intermittent fasting is for those who want to regulate their hormones and burn surplus body fat. This diet allows for healthier whole foods and an all-round diet, which is better than living off processed foods and sugars, which are unhealthy. It can also benefit individuals who are sugar-addicted or those who ate empty calories. Drinks and sodas with very few nutrients, but full of calories, are included in these products. Finally, people generally want to do better in life and enjoy a food plan that doesn't require too much planning or maintenance.

Even if intermittent fasting may not be for you reading this book will equip you with the necessary information required to help another person or to use it eventually in life.

Different Methods

IF regiments are numerous to the point that you can choose from any that you like. Always make sure to select a regimen that will fit in your schedule so that it is possible to maintain it.

There are several short methods for fasting, including:

The 12-Hour Fast

That's what the regular living routine is called as you eat three meals a day and fast at night as you sleep. The generally small breakfast would break the fast. It is called the traditional method. Any regiment can help you lose weight only if you follow it correctly.

The higher the levels of insulin are as a result of more people adding regular eating and snacking. It can cause resistance to insulin and, ultimately, obesity. This fasting technique sets aside twelve hours in which the body has low insulin levels, reducing the likelihood of insulin resistance. It can't help you lose excess fat, but it can help prevent obesity.

The 16-Hour Fast

This fasting for 16 hours is followed by an 8-hour window where you can eat what you like. Luckily you can sleep through most of it, so it's not difficult to keep doing it. Because it requires only small changes like just skipping your lunch, it has an enormous advantage over others, such as the 12 hours fast.

The 20-Hour Fast

It's called the "warrior diet." It includes fasting all day long and eating a lot of calories at night. It's meant to keep you from having breakfast, lunch, and other meals for most of the day, so you're getting all your nutrients from dinner. It is a division scheme of 20:4 with four hours of food followed by twenty hours of fasting. It's one of the easiest to do as you're allowed to eat a huge meal of calorific value, so you're going to feel fuller for longer. Start your daytime calories and have a big evening dinner to relax in this diet. You're going to gradually reduce what you're eating during the day and eventually leave dinner as your only meal.

The longer you do these fasting regiments, the more you will be able to maintain a fast. You will come to find out that you will not always feel hungry. The excitement of benefits will make you increase your period of fasting by a couple of hours. Unknowingly, therefore, you are plunging into longer stages of fasting. You can adhere to your regiment religiously, but eating an extra hour will not ruin your fasting or fat burning.

The easiest way to track your feeding is to do it once a day is because it doesn't require a lot of thought. It's just eating at that moment every day on one dinner so that you can use your mental energy on the more important stuff. Unfortunately, it can cause a plateau of weight loss, where you are not losing or gaining weight.

That's because you're going to consume the same number of calories every day and significantly less on a typical working day than you would eat. That's the best way to maintain your weight. You will have to change your fasting regiment to lose fat after a while. Timing your meals and fasting windows will lead to optimal loss of fat instead of random fasting. Choose one that can be maintained and modified if necessary.

There are longer fasting regiments, these include:

The 24-Hour Fast

It's a scheme of eating breakfast, lunch, or dinner in a day and then eating the following day at the same time. If you decide to eat lunch, then it only involves skipping breakfast and dinner, so nothing is disrupted in your life. It saves time and money because you're not going to eat as much, and piling up dishes will not be a worry of yours. Knowing that you are fasting will be a task for people unless they are very interested in eating methods. By eating unprocessed natural foods, you should have enough vitamins, minerals, and oxygen to avoid nutrient deficiencies. You can do this weekly, but twice or three times a week, it is suggested.

During such long fasts, you should not knowingly avoid eating calories. What you are taking should be high in fat, low in carbohydrates, and unprocessed; there's nothing you shouldn't eat. It would be best if you consumed until you are adequately fed as the duration of fasting lets you burn a bunch of fat, and it will be difficult over time to try to cut more purposefully.

The 36-Hour Fast

You retain in this fast for one and a half days without eating. For instance, if you eat lunch today, you consume no meal until the day's breakfast after the following day. This fast should be done about three times a week for people with type 2 diabetes. After the person reaches the desired weight and all diabetes medications are successfully removed, they can reduce the number of days of fasting to a level that will make it easier for them to do while maintaining their gains. Blood sugar should usually be checked as small or high.

The 42-Hour Fast

It is adding six hours to the 36 hours fast, resulting in a fast of forty-two hours carried out about two times a week.

The 5:2 Fast

This technique is conducted to prevent you from totally abstaining from meals and have cycles of calorie consumption. These calories are reduced to a rate that leads to many hormonal advantages of fasting. It consists of five days of regular feeding with two days of fasting. With some protein and oil-based sauce or green vegetables and half an avocado, you can eat some vegetable salad during these fasting days; furthermore, do not eat any dinner. These days of fasting can be placed randomly or following each other in a week at specific times. This method is designed to create faster for more people, as many find it challenging to avoid eating altogether. There's no exact time to follow; as soon as you want, you can follow it.

The Alternate-Day Fast

It may seem similar to the 5:2 fasting regimen, but it is not. It's fasting every day. This technique can be followed until you lose as much weight as you want, then you can reduce days of fasting. It allows weight loss to be maintained.

It is possible to move to different fasting regiments as your schedule can change. Intermittent fasting is not about a time-limiting eating window; it is flexible, so you can move your eating and fasting time to suit you, but don't keep changing them all the time; this reduces the effect of fasting on your body. You can even combine some fasting regiments like the 5:2 technique and the 24-hour fasting by having lunch before your fasting day at a particular moment and adding only lunch at the fasting lunch and doing the same for the following fasting day. With this, for twenty-four hours, you could not eat any calories and set your days of fasting as in the 5:2 method of fasting. Choose the fasting day technique that works well with you and can synchronize with your life.

A schedule allows you to create a routine after frequent fasting that makes it easier to integrate into your life. You can plan, but there's no problem if you can't. Even if you can't plan to fast, you should be open-minded fasting to opportunities. You can fast every month or every year. Frankly, you won't lose weight on losing annual fasts.

Intermittent and Keto Diet

You know all of the different ways to fast, and you know what the ketogenic diet is. The primary purpose of intermittent fasting is to not eat as much during the day. Intermittent fasting can boost your fat burning. When your body is a fasted state, your body will turn to your fat stores for energy. It is when the body starts forming ketones to fuel you and your brain. Now, the ketogenic diet does the same thing without any fasting. However, many people find they don't feel as hungry when following a keto diet. It means that they start fasting simply because they don't feel like they need to eat.

You don't have to fast when on keto, and you don't have to follow keto when fasting. You can choose whichever method, but some people will find that fasting becomes easier on a ketogenic diet.

People who follow a ketogenic diet will have lower insulin levels and blood glucose levels. They have a reduced appetite because of the effects of the ketogenic diet. It means that they won't have any sugar crashes, and they won't feel as hungry.

If you maintain a regular diet, high in carbs, and fasting, you may experience an increase in hunger hormones, and your blood glucose may drop quickly. It could end up causing you to feel irritable, shaky, and weak. It could mean that you feel hungry all of the time. It doesn't always happen, though.

Using both ketogenic diet and intermittent fasting for weight loss is a great idea, but remember, you can use them separately.

FOOD LIST-What to Eat and Avoid

I've had people complain about the difficulty of switching their grocery list to one that's Ketogenic-friendly. The fact is that food is expensive, and most of the food you have in your fridge is probably packed full of carbohydrates. It is why if you're committing to a Ketogenic Diet, you need to do a clean sweep. That's right, everything that's packed with carbohydrates should be identified and set aside to make sure that you are not overeating.

What to Eat on the Keto Diet

Fats and Oils

Because fats will be included as part of all your meals, we recommend that you choose the highest quality ingredients that you can afford. Some of your best choices for fat are:

- Ghee or Clarified butter
- Avocado
- Coconut Oil
- Red Palm Oil
- Butter
- Coconut Butter
- Peanut Butter
- Chicken Fat
- Beef Tallow
- Non-hydrogenated Lard
- Macadamias and other nuts
- Egg Yolks
- Fish rich in Omega-3 Fatty Acids like salmon, mackerel, trout, tuna, and shellfish

Protein

Those on a keto diet will generally keep fat intake high, carbohydrate intake low, and protein intake at a moderate level. Some on the keto diet for weight loss have better success with higher protein and lower fat intake.

- **Fresh meat:** beef, veal, lamb, chicken, duck, pheasant, pork, etc.
- **·Deli meats:** bacon, sausage, ham (make sure to watch out for added sugar and other fillers)
- **Eggs:** preferably free-range or organic eggs
- **Fish:** wild-caught salmon, catfish, halibut, trout, tuna, etc.
- **Other seafood:** lobster, crab, oyster, clams, mussels, etc.
- **Peanut Butter:** this is a great source of protein, but make sure to choose a brand that contains no added sugar

Dairy

Compared to other weight-loss diets, the keto diet actually encourages you to choose dairy products that are full fat. Some of the best dairy products that you can choose are:

- ·Hard and soft cheese: cream cheese, mozzarella, cheddar, etc.
- ·Cottage cheese
- ·Heavy whipping cream
- ·Sour cream
- ·Full-fat yogurt

Vegetables

Overall, vegetables are rich in vitamins and minerals that contribute to a healthy body. However, if you're aiming to avoid carbs, it's best that you limit starchy vegetables such as potatoes, yams, peas, corn, beans, and most legumes. Other vegetables that are high in carbohydrates, such as parsnips and squash, should also be limited. Instead, stick with green leafy vegetables and other low-carb veggies. Choose local or organic varieties if it fits with your budget.

- ·Spinach
- ·Lettuce
- ·Collard greens
- ·Mustard greens
- ·Bok choy
- ·Kale

- Alfalfa sprouts
- Celery
- Tomato
- Broccoli
- Cauliflower
- Fruits

- Your choice of fruit on the keto diet is typically restricted to avocado and berries because fruits are high in carbohydrates and sugar.
- Drinks
- ·Water
- ·Black coffee
- ·Herbal tea
- ·Wine: white wine and dry red wine are OK if they are only consumed occasionally.

Others

- Homemade mayo: if you want to buy mayo from the store, make sure that you watch out for added sugar
- Homemade mustard
- Any type of spices or herbs
- Stevia and other non-nutritive sweeteners such as Swerve
- Ketchup (Sugar-free)
- Dark chocolate/cocoa

Foods to Avoid

1. Bread and Grains

Bread is a staple food in many countries. You have loaves, bagels, tortillas, and the list goes on. However, no matter what form bread takes, they still contain a lot of carbs. The same applies to whole-grain as well because they are made from refined flour. Depending on your daily carb limit, eating a sandwich or bagel can put your way over your daily limit. So if you want to eat bread, it is best to make keto variants at home instead. Grains such as rice, wheat, and oats contain a lot of carbs too. So limit or avoid that as well.

1. Fruits

Fruits are healthy for you. They are found to make you have a lower risk of heart disease and cancer. However, there are a few that you need to avoid in your keto diet. The problem is that some of those foods contain quite a lot of carbs, such as banana, raisins, dates, mango, and pear. As a general rule, avoid sweet and dried fruits. Berries are an exception because they do not contain as much sugar and are rich in fiber. So you can still eat some of them, around 50 grams. Moderation is key.

2. Vegetables

Vegetables are healthy for your body. Most of the keto diet does not care how many vegetables you eat so long as they are low in starch. Vegetables that are high in fiber can aid with weight loss..

On the one hand, they make you feel full for longer, so they help suppress your appetite. Another benefit is that your body would burn more calories to break and digest them.

Moreover, they help control blood sugar levels and aid with your bowel movements. But that also means you need to avoid or limit vegetables that are high in starch because they have more carbs than fiber. That includes corn, potato, sweet potato, and beets.

1. Pasta

Pasta is also a staple food in many countries. It is versatile and convenient. As with any other suitable food, pasta is rich in carbs. So when you are on your keto diet, spaghetti, or many different types of pasta are not recommended. You can probably eat a small portion, but that is not suggested. Thankfully, that does not mean you need to give up on it altogether. If you are craving pasta, you can try some other alternatives that are low in carbs such as spiralized veggies or shirataki noodles.

2. Cereal

Cereal is also a massive offender because sugary breakfast cereals contain a lot of carbs. That also applies to "healthy cereals." Just because they use other words to describe their product does not mean that you should believe them. That also applies to oatmeal, whole-grain cereals, etc. So if you get your cereal when you are doing keto, you are already way over your carb limit, and we haven't even added milk into the equation! Therefore, avoid whole-grain cereal or cereals that we mention here altogether.

Health Tips for People After 50

Nobody told you that life was going to be this way! But don't worry. There's still plenty of time to make amendments and take care of your health. Here are a couple of tips that will allow you to lead a healthier life in your fifties:

Start Building on Immunity

Every day, our body is exposed to free radicals and toxins from the environment. The added stress of work and family problems doesn't make it any easier for us. To combat this, you must start consuming healthy veggies that contain plenty of antioxidants and build a healthier immune system.

This helps ward off unwanted illnesses and diseases, allowing you to maintain good health.

Adding more healthy veggies to your keto diet will help you obtain various minerals, vitamins, and antioxidants.

Consider Quitting Smoking

It's never too late to try to quit smoking, even if you are in your fifties. Once a smoker begins to quit, the body quickly starts to heal the previous damages caused by smoking.

Once you start quitting, you'll notice how you'll be able to breathe easier while acquiring a better sense of smell and taste. Over a period of time, eliminating the habit of smoking can greatly reduce the risks of high blood pressure, strokes, and heart attack. Please note how these diseases are much more common among people in the fifties and above than in younger people.

Not to mention, quitting smoking will help you stay more active and enjoy better health with your friends and family.

Stay Social

We've already mentioned this, but it's worth pondering on again and again. Aging can be a daunting process, and trying to get through it all on your own isn't particularly helpful. We recommend you to stay in touch with friends and family or become a part of a local community club or network. Some older people find it comforting to get an emotional support animal.

Being surrounded by people you love will give you a sense of belonging and will improve your mood. It'll also keep your mind and memory sharp as you engage in different conversations.

Health Screenings You Should Get After Your Fifties

Your fifties are considered the prime years of your life. Don't let the joy of these years be robbed away from you because of poor health. Getting simple tests done can go a long way in identifying any potential health problems that you may have. Here is a list of health screenings you should get done:

Check Your Blood Pressure

Your blood pressure is a reliable indicator of your heart health. In simple words, blood pressure is a measure of how fast blood travels through the artery walls. Very high or even very low blood pressure can be a sign of an underlying problem. Once you reach your 40s, you should have your blood pressure checked more often.

EKG

The EKG reveals your heart health and activity. Short for electrocardiogram, the EKG helps identify problems in the heart.

The process works by highlighting any rhythm problems that may be in the heart, such as poor heart muscles, improper blood flow, or any other form of abnormality. Getting an EKG is also a predictive measure for understanding the chances of a heart attack. Since people starting their fifties are at greater risk of getting a heart attack, you should get yourself checked more often.

Mammogram

Mammograms help rule out the risks of breast cancer. Women who enter their fifties should ideally get a mammogram after every ten years. However, if you have a family history, it is advisable that you get one much earlier to rule out cancer possibilities.

Blood Sugar Levels

If you're somebody who used to grab a fast food meal every once in a while before you switched to keto, then you should definitely check your blood sugar levels more carefully. Blood sugar levels indicate whether or not you have diabetes. And you know how the saying goes, "prevention is better than cure." It's best to clear these possibilities out of the way sooner than later.

Check for Osteoporosis

Unfortunately, as you grow older, you also become susceptible to a number of bone diseases. Osteoporosis is a bone-related condition in which bones begin to lose mass, becoming frail and weak. Owing to this, seniors become more prone to fractures. This can make even the smallest of falls detrimental to your health.

Annual Physical Exam

Your insurance must be providing coverage for your annual physical exam. So, there's no reason why you should not take advantage of it. This checkup helps identify the state of your health. You'll probably be surprised by how much doctors can tell from a single blood test.

Prostate Screening Exam

Once men hit their fifties, they should be screened for prostate cancer (similar to how women should get a mammogram and pap smear). Getting a screening done becomes especially important if cancer runs in your family.

Eye Exam

As you start to aging, you'll notice how your eyesight will start to deteriorate. It's quite likely that vision is not as sharp as it used to be. Ideally, you should have gotten your first eye exam during your 40s, but it isn't too late. Get one as soon as possible to prevent symptoms from escalating.

Be Wary of Any Weird Moles

While skin cancer can become a problem at any age, older adults should pay closer attention to any moles or unusual skin tags in their bodies. While most cancers can be easily treated, melanoma can be particularly quite dangerous. If you have noticed any recent moles in your body that have changed in color, size, or shape, make sure to visit the dermatologist.

Check Your Cholesterol Levels

We've talked about this plenty of times, but it's worth mentioning again. High cholesterol levels can be dangerous to your health and can be an indicator of many diseases. Things become more complicated for conditions that don't show particular symptoms. Your total cholesterol levels should be below 200 mg per deciliter just to be on the safe side. Your doctor will take a simple blood test and will give you a couple of guidelines with the results. In case there is something to be worried about, you should make serious dietary and lifestyle changes.

Within the first few weeks, just about everyone who follows this program experiences a rapid and significant weight loss. I've had readers tell me they've lost about 14 pounds in 14 days. These outcomes vary from person to person. If you have much extra weight to lose, it's likely to come off quicker. Some of the weight loss will be water weight, and it will feel right that the scale is going down fast. It may get you motivated to continue.

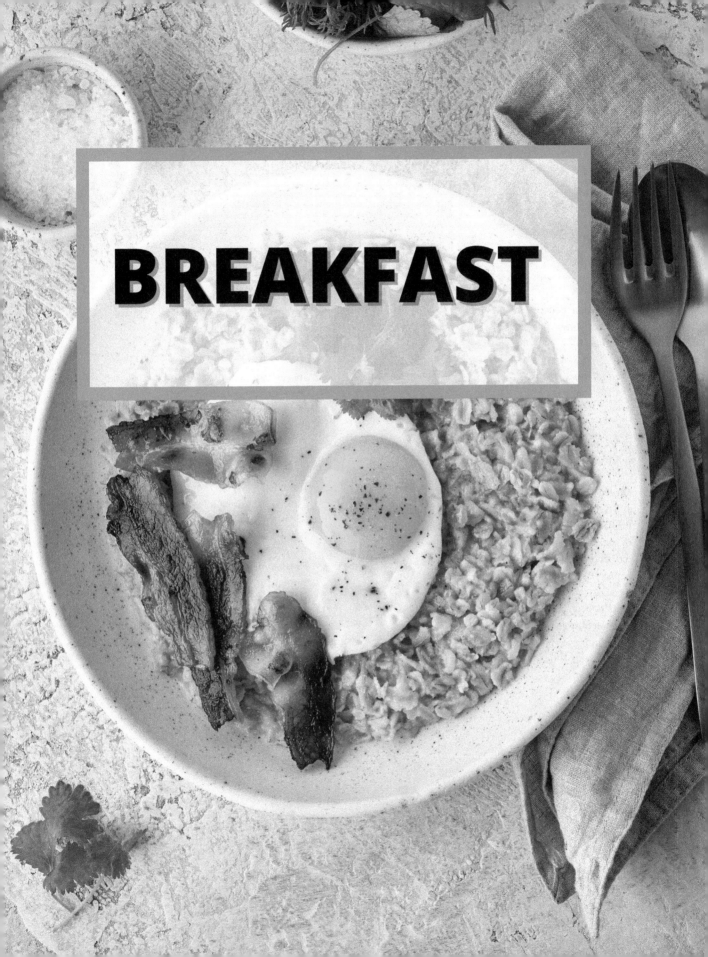

BREAKFAST

1. Cheesy Bacon & Egg Cups

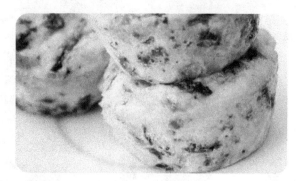

Preparation Time: 10 minutes
Cooking Time: 20 minutes
Servings: 6

·**Ingredients:**
- 6 bacon slices
- 6 large eggs
- .25 cup cheese
- 1 spinach
- Pepper

Directions:
1. Set the oven setting to 400º Fahrenheit (204ºC). Cook the bacon in medium-heat. Grease muffin tins. Put the slice of bacon. Mix the eggs and combine with the spinach. Add the batter to tins and sprinkle with cheese. Put salt and pepper. Bake for 15 minutes. Serve.

Nutrition:
Carbohydrate: 1 gram
Protein: 8 grams
Fat: 7 grams
Calories: 101

2. Coconut Keto Porridge

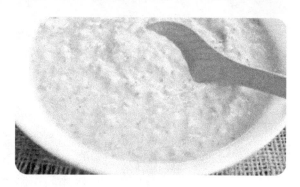

Preparation Time: 15 minutes
Cooking Time: 10 minutes
Servings: 1

Ingredients:
- 4tsp. coconut cream
- 1 pinch ground psyllium husk powder
- 1 tbsp. coconut flour
- 1 Flaxseed egg
- 1 oz. coconut butter

Directions:
Toss all of the mixture in a small pan, cook on low heat. Serve.

Nutrition:
Carbohydrate: 5.4 grams
Protein: 10.1 grams
Fat: 22.8 grams
Calories: 401

3. Cream Cheese Eggs

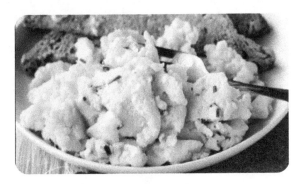

Preparation Time: 5 minutes
Cooking Time: 5 minutes
Servings: 1

Ingredients:
- 1 tbsp. butter
- 2 eggs
- 2 tbsp. soft cream cheese with chives

Directions:
1. Heat a skillet and melt the butter. Whisk the eggs with the cream cheese.
2. Cook until done. Serve.

Nutrition:
Carbohydrate: 3 grams
Protein: 15 grams
Fat: 31 grams
Calories: 341

4. Creamy Basil Baked Sausage

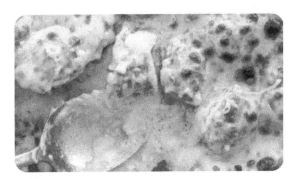

Preparation Time: 5 minutes
Cooking Time: 30-40 minutes
Servings: 12

Ingredients:
- 3 lb. (1.3 kg.) Italian sausage
- 8 oz. cream cheese
- 25 cup heavy cream
- .25 cup basil pesto
- 8 oz. mozzarella

Directions:
1. Set the oven at 400º Fahrenheit.
2. Put the sausage to the dish and bake for 30 minutes. Combine the heavy cream, pesto, and cream cheese. Pour the sauce over the casserole and top it off with the cheese.
3. Bake for 10 minutes. Serve.

Nutrition:
Carbohydrate: 4 grams
Protein: 23 grams
Fat: 23 grams
Calories: 316

5. Almond Coconut Egg Wraps

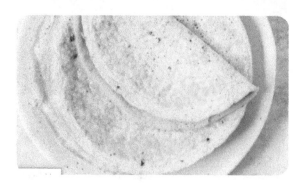

Preparation Time: 5 minutes
Cooking Time: 5 minutes
Servings: 4

Ingredients:
- 5 organic eggs
- 1 tbsp. coconut flour
- .25 tsp. sea salt
- 2 tbsp. almond meal

Directions:
1. Put the mixture in a blender. Warm-up a skillet, medium-high. Add two tablespoons of batter then cook for 3 minutes. Flip to cook for another 3 minutes. Serve.

Nutrition:
Carbohydrate: 3 grams
Protein: 8 grams
Fat: 8 grams
Calories: 111

6. Ricotta Cloud Pancakes

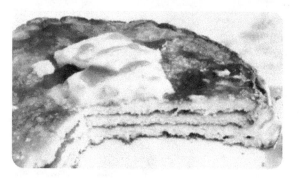

Preparation Time: 10 minutes
Cooking Time: 2 minutes
Servings: 4

Ingredients:
- 1 cup almond flour
- 1 tsp low carb baking powder
- 2 ½ tbsp swerve
- 1/3 tsp salt
- 1 ¼ cup ricotta cheese
- 1/3 cup coconut milk
- 2 large eggs
- 1 cup heavy whipping cream

Directions:
1. In a medium bowl, whisk the almond flour, baking powder, swerve, and salt. Set aside.
2. Then, crack the eggs into the blender and process on medium speed for 30 seconds. Add the ricotta cheese, continue processing it, and gradually pour the coconut milk in while you keep on blending.
3. In about 90 seconds, the mixture will be creamy and smooth. Pour it into the dry ingredients and whisk to combine.
4. Set a skillet over medium heat and let it heat for a minute. Then, pour a soup spoonful of mixture into the skillet and cook for 1 minute.
5. Flip the pancake and cook further for 1 minute. Serve on a plate and repeat the cooking process until the batter is exhausted. Serve the pancakes with whipping cream.

Nutrition:
Carbohydrate: 7g
Fat: 31g
Protein: 12g
Calories: 407

7. Keto Cinnamon Coffee

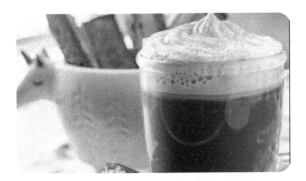

Preparation Time: 5 minutes
Cooking Time: 5 minutes
Servings: 1

Ingredients:
- 2tbsp. ground coffee
- 1/3 cup heavy whipping cream
- 1tsp. ground cinnamon
- 2 cups of water

Directions:
1. Start by mixing the cinnamon with the ground coffee. Pour in hot water, whip the cream until stiff peaks. Serve with cinnamon.

Nutrition:
Carbohydrate: 1g
Fiber: 1g
Fat: 14g
Protein: 1g
Calories: 136

8. Keto Waffles and Blueberries

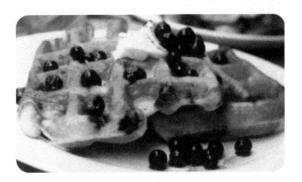

Preparation Time: 15 minutes
Cooking Time: 10 to 15 minutes
Servings: 8

Ingredients:
- 8 eggs
- 5 oz. (141 g) melted butter
- 1 tsp. vanilla extract
- 2 tsp. baking powder
- 1/3 cup coconut flour
- Topping:
- 3 oz. (85 g) butter
- 1 oz. (28 g) blueberries

Directions:
1. Mix the butter and eggs, put in the remaining items except topping.
2. Cook the batter in medium heat. Serve with blueberries.

Nutrition:
Carbohydrate: 3g
Fiber: 5g
Fat: 56g
Protein: 14g
Calories: 575

9. Baked Avocado Eggs

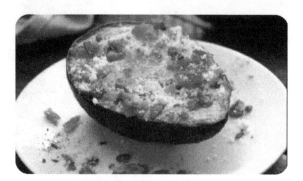

Preparation Time: 30 minutes
Cooking Time: 30 minutes
Servings: 4

Ingredients:
- avocados
- 4 eggs
- ½ cup bacon bits
- 2 tbsp. chives
- 1 sprig basil
- 1 cherry tomato
- Salt
- pepper
- Shredded cheddar cheese

Directions:
Heat the oven to 400 degrees Fahrenheit (204ºC).
Remove the avocado seed. Break eggs onto the center hole of the avocado. Put salt and pepper.
Top with bacon bits and bake for 15 minutes. Serve!

Nutrition:
Calories: 271
Fat: 21g
Fiber: 5g
Protein: 13g
Carbohydrate: 7g.

10. Mushroom Omelet

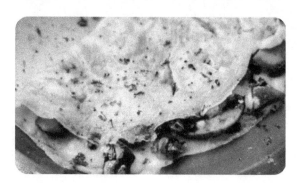

Preparation Time: 15 minutes
Cooking Time: 5 minutes
Servings: 1

Ingredients:
- 3 eggs
- 1 oz. (28 g) cheese
- 1 oz. (28 g) butter
- ¼ yellow onion
- 4 large mushrooms
- vegetables
- Salt
- pepper

Directions:
1. Beat the eggs, put some salt and pepper.
2. Cook the mushroom and onion. Put the egg mixture into the pan and cook on medium heat.
3. Put the cheese on top of the still-raw portion of the egg.
4. Pry the edges of the omelet and fold it in half. Serve.

Nutrition:
Carbohydrate: 5g
Fiber: 1g
Fat: 44g
Protein: 26g
Calories: 520

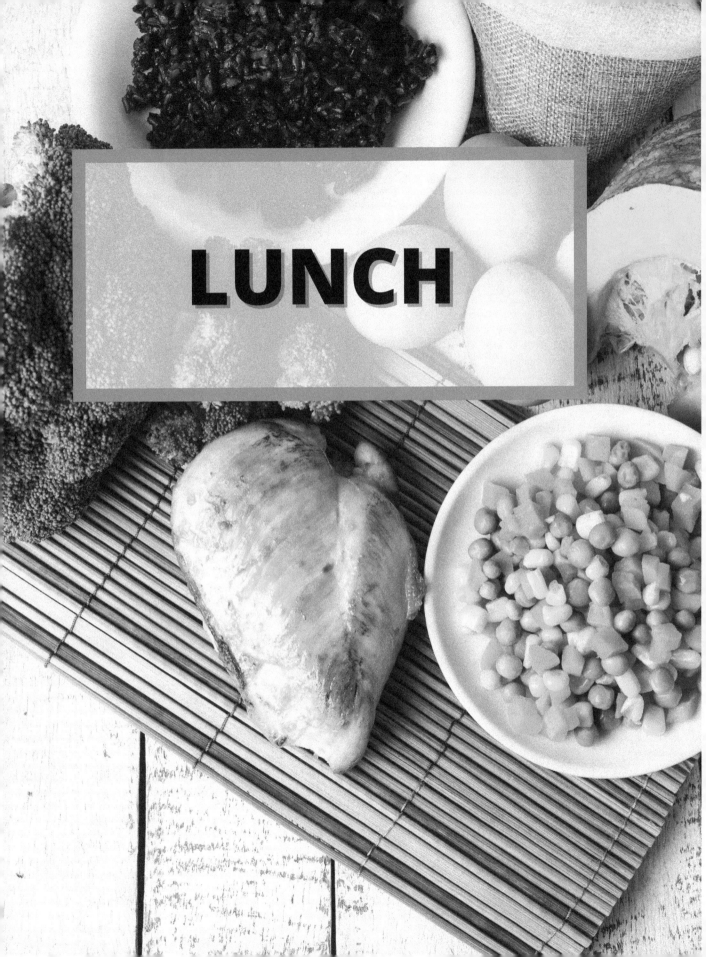

11. Loaded Cauliflower Salad

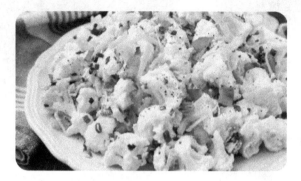

Preparation Time: 15 minutes
Cooking Time: 30 minutes
Servings: 4

Ingredients:
- One large head cauliflower
- Six slices bacon
- ½ c. sour cream
- ¼ c. mayonnaise
- 1 tbsp. lemon juice
- ½ tsp. garlic powder
- Kosher salt
- Ground black pepper
- 1 ½ c. cheddar
- ¼ c. chives

Directions:
1. Boil ¼ water, put cauliflower, cover pan, and steam for 4 minutes. Drain and cool.
2. Cook the pork around 3 minutes per side. Drain then cut.
3. Mix the sour cream, mayonnaise, lemon juice, and garlic powder in a big bowl. Toss the cauliflower florets. Put salt pepper, bacon, cheddar, and chives. Serve.

Nutrition:
Carbohydrate: 13g
Fiber: 4g
Fat: 25g
Protein: 19g
Calories: 440

12. Caprese Zoodles

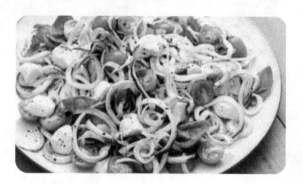

Preparation Time: 15 minutes
Cooking Time: 0 minutes
Servings: 4

Ingredients:
- Four zucchinis
- 2 tbsp. extra-virgin olive oil
- Kosher salt
- Ground black pepper
- 2 c. cherry tomatoes halved
- 1 c. mozzarella balls
- ¼ c. basil leaves
- 2 tbsp. balsamic vinegar

Directions:
1. Creating zoodles out of zucchini using a spiralizer.
1. Mix the zoodles, olive oil, salt, and pepper. Marinate for 15 minutes.
2. Put the tomatoes, mozzarella, and basil and toss.
3. Drizzle, and drink with balsamic.

Nutrition:
Carbohydrate: 11g
Fiber: 4gr
Fat: 24g
Protein: 36g
Calories: 417

13. Zucchini Sushi

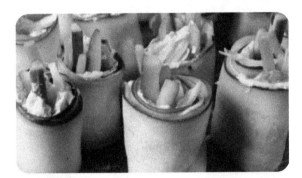

Preparation Time: 20 minutes
Cooking Time: 0 minutes
Servings: 6

Ingredients:
- Two zucchinis
- 4 oz. (113 g) cream cheese
- 1 tsp. sriracha hot sauce
- 1 tsp. lime juice
- 1 c. lump crab meat
- ½ carrot
- ½ avocado
- ½ cucumber
- 1 tsp. toasted sesame seeds

Directions:
· Slice each zucchini into thin flat strips. Put aside.
· Combine cream cheese, sriracha, and lime juice in a medium-sized cup.
· Place two slices of zucchini horizontally flat on a cutting board. Place a lean layer of cream cheese over it, then top the left with a slice of lobster, carrot, avocado, and cucumber.
· Roll up zucchini. Serve with sesame seeds.

Nutrition:
Carbohydrate: 23g
Fiber: 5g
Fat: 25g
Protein: 35g
Calories: 450

14. Chicken Tacos

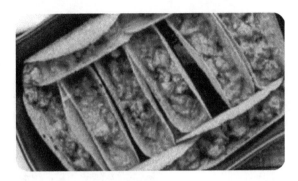

Preparation Time: 15 minutes
Cooking Time: 20 minutes
Servings: 4

Ingredients:
- 1 pound (453 g) ground chicken
- 1 ½ cups Mexican cheese blend
- 1 tablespoon Mexican seasoning blend
- 2 teaspoons butter, room temperature
- 2 small-sized shallots, peeled and finely chopped
- 1 clove garlic, minced
- 1 cup tomato puree
- 1/2 cup salsa
- 2 slices bacon, chopped

Directions:
1. Melt the butter in a saucepan over moderately high flame. Now, cook the shallots until tender and fragrant.
2. Then, sauté the garlic, chicken, and bacon for about 5 minutes, stirring continuously and crumbling with a fork. Add the in Mexican seasoning blend.
3. Add the tomato puree and salsa; continue to simmer for 5 to 7 minutes over medium-low heat; reserve.
4. Line a baking pan with wax paper. Place 4 piles of the shredded cheese on the baking pan and gently press them down with a wide spatula to make "taco shells".
5. Bake in the preheated oven at 365 degrees F (185°C) for 6 to 7 minutes or until melted. Allow these taco shells to cool for about 10 minutes.

Nutrition:
Carbohydrate: 28g
Fat: 3g
Protein: 24g
Calories: 260

15. California Burger Bowls

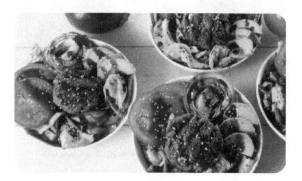

Preparation Time: 15 minutes
Cooking Time: 20 minutes
Servings: 4

Ingredients:

For the dressing:
- ½ c. extra-virgin olive oil
- 1/3 c. balsamic vinegar
- 3 tbsp. Dijon mustard
- 2 tsp. honey
- One clove garlic
- Kosher salt
- Ground black pepper

For the burger:
- 1 lb. (453 g) grass-fed organic ground beef
- 1 tsp. Worcestershire sauce
- ½ tsp. chili powder
- ½ tsp. onion powder
- Kosher salt
- Ground black pepper
- One package butterhead lettuce
- One medium red onion
- One avocado
- 2 tomatoes

Directions:

Make the dressing:
1. Mix the dressing items in a medium bowl.

Make burgers:
1. Combine beef and Worcestershire sauce, chili powder, and onion powder in another large bowl. Put pepper and salt, mix. Form into four patties.
2. Grill the onions for 3 minutes each. Remove and detach burgers from the grill pan. Cook for 4 minutes per side.

Assemble:
3. Put lettuce in a large bowl with ½ the dressing. Finish with a patty burger, grilled onions, ¼ slices of avocado, and tomatoes. Serve.

Nutrition:
Calories: 407
Carbohydrate: 33g
Fat: 19g
Protein: 26g

16. Parmesan Brussels Sprouts Salad

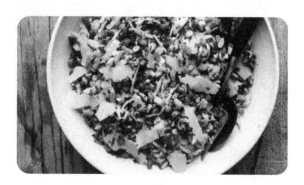

Preparation Time: 15 minutes
Cooking Time: 25 minutes
Servings: 6

Ingredients:
- 5 tbsp. extra-virgin olive oil
- 5 tbsp. lemon juice
- ¼ c. parsley
- Kosher salt
- Ground black pepper
- 2 lb. Brussels sprouts
- ½ c. toasted almonds
- ½ c. pomegranate seeds
- Shaved Parmesan

Directions:
1. Mix olive oil, lemon juice, parsley, two teaspoons of salt, and one teaspoon of pepper.
1. Add the sprouts in Brussels and toss.
2. Let sit before serving for 20 minutes and up to 4 hours.
3. Fold in almonds and pomegranate seeds and garnish with a rasped parmesan. Serve.

Nutrition:
Calories: 130
Carbohydrate: 8g
Fat: 9g
Protein: 4g

17. Shrimp and Avocado Lettuce

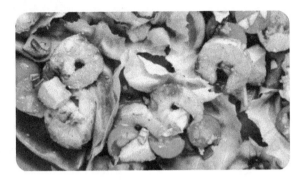

Preparation Time: 10 minutes
Cooking Time: 5 minutes
Servings: 2

Ingredients:
- 1 tablespoon ghee
- ½ pound shrimp
- ½ cup halved grape tomatoes
- ½ avocado, sliced
- 4 butter lettuce leaves, rinsed and patted dry

Directions:
1. In a medium skillet put the ghee at medium-high heat. Add the shrimp and cook. Season with pink salt and pepper. Shrimp are cooked when they turn pink and opaque.
2. Season the tomatoes and avocado with pink salt and pepper. Divide the lettuce cups between two plates. Fill each cup with shrimp, tomatoes, and avocado. Drizzle the mayo sauce on top and serve.

Nutrition:
Calories: 324
Carbohydrate: 16g
Fat: 24g
Protein: 15g

18. Keto Quesadillas

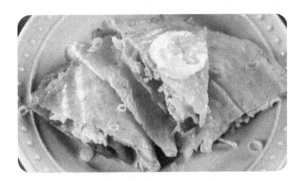

Preparation Time: 15 minutes
Cooking Time: 25 minutes
Servings: 4
Ingredients:
- 1 tbsp. extra-virgin olive oil
- One bell pepper
- ½ yellow onion
- ½ tsp. chili powder
- Kosher salt
- Ground black pepper
- 3 c. Monterey Jack
- 3 c. cheddar
- 4 c. chicken
- One avocado
- One green onion
- Sour cream

Directions:
· Heat the oven to 400 F (204ºC). Line two medium parchment paper baking sheets.
· Heat oil in a medium skillet. Put the onion and pepper, chili powder, salt, and pepper. Cook for 5 minutes.
· Stir cheeses in a medium-sized dish. Put 1 ½ cups of mixed cheese to prepared baking sheets. Form a circle, the size of a tortilla flour.
· Bake the cheeses for 8 to 10 minutes. Put a batter of onion-pepper, shredded chicken, and slices of avocado to one half each. Cool and fold one side of the "tortilla" cheese over the side with the fillings. Bake for 3 to 4 more minutes.
· Serve with green onion and sour cream.
Nutrition:
Calories: 473
Carbohydrate: 5g
Fat: 41g
Protein: 21g

19. No-Bread Italian Subs

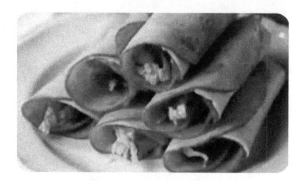

Preparation Time: 15 minutes
Cooking Time: 15 minutes
Servings: 6

Ingredients:
- ½ c. mayonnaise
- 2 tbsp.red wine vinegar
- 1 tbsp. extra-virgin olive oil
- One small garlic clove, grated
- 1 tsp. Italian seasoning
- Six slices ham
- 12 salami slices
- 12 pepperoni slices
- Six provolone slices
- 1 c. romaine
- ½ c. roasted red peppers

Directions:
1. Make creamy Italian dressing:
1. Mix the mayo, vinegar, butter, garlic, and Italian seasoning.
2. Assemble sandwiches:
3. Stack a ham slice, two salami pieces, two pepperoni slices, and a provolone slice.
4. Put a handful of romaine and a couple of roasted red peppers. Put creamy Italian sauce, then roll in and eat.

Nutrition:
Calories: 390;
Protein: 16g
Carbohydrate: 3g;
Fat: 34g

20. Turkey Meatballs

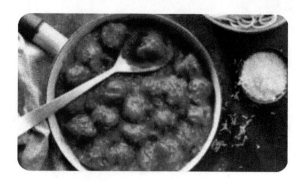

Preparation Time: 15 minutes
Cooking Time: 10 minutes
Servings: 4

Ingredients:
For the Meatballs:
- 1/3 cup Colby cheese, freshly grated
- 3/4 pound (340 g) ground turkey
- 1/3 teaspoon Five-spice powder
- 1 egg
- For the Sauce:
- 1 1/3 cups water
- 1/3 cup champagne vinegar
- 2 tablespoons soy sauce
- 1/2 cup Swerve
- 1/2 cup tomato sauce, no sugar added
- 1/2 teaspoon paprika
- 1/3 teaspoon guar gum

Directions:
1. Thoroughly combine all ingredients for the meatballs. Roll the mixture into balls and sear them until browned on all sides.
2. In a saucepan, mix all of the sauce ingredients and cook until the sauce has thickened, whisking continuously.
3. Fold the meatballs into the sauce and continue to cook, partially covered, for about 10 minutes.

Nutrition:
Calories: 160
Carbs: 6g
Fat: 9g
Protein: 14g

21. Cauliflower Leek Soup

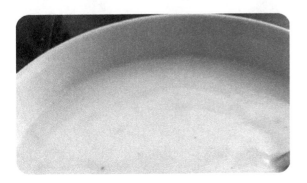

Preparation Time: 15 minutes
Cooking Time: 50 minutes
Servings: 2

Ingredients:
- ½ tablespoons olive oil
- ½ tablespoon garlic
- ½ tablespoons butter
- 2 cups Vegetable Broth
- 1 leek
- Salt
- 1 cup cauliflower
- black pepper
- ¼ cup heavy cream

Directions:
Put the oil and butter in the pan to heat. Add garlic, cauliflower, and leek pieces and cook for 5 minutes on low.
· Add vegetable broth and boil. Cover the pan and cook on low for 45 minutes.
· Remove then blend the soup in a mixer. Put heavy cream, salt, pepper, and blend more.
· Serve with salt and pepper.

Nutrition:
Calories: 155 kcal
Fat: 13.1 g
Carbohydrate: 8.3 g
Protein: 2.4 g

22. Sugar-Free Blueberry Cottage Cheese Parfaits

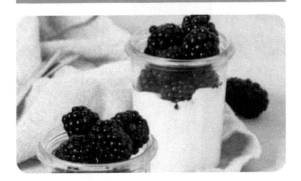

Preparation Time: 5 minutes
Cooking Time: 5 minutes
Servings: 2

Ingredients:
- 0.5 pounds (225 g) cheese, low fat
- 1/8 tablespoon cinnamon
- ¼ vanilla extract
- 6 drops stevia, liquid
- 0.33 pounds (150 g) berries

Directions:
1. Blend cheese, vanilla extract, cinnamon, and stevia into the blender.
1. Remove and pour these into bowls.
2. Put the berries on top of the cheese parfaits. Serve.

Nutrition:
Calories: 125 kcal
Fat: 2.2 g
Carbohydrate: 12.5 g
Protein: 14.8g
Fiber: 1.5 g

23. Low-Calorie Cheesy Broccoli Quiche

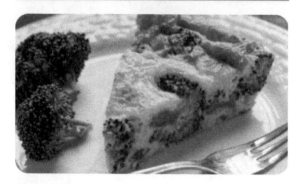

Preparation Time: 25 minutes
Cooking Time: 30 minutes
Servings: 2

Ingredients:
- 1/3 tablespoon butter
- Black pepper
- 4 oz. broccoli
- ¼ teaspoon garlic powder
- 2 tablespoon full-fat cream
- 1/8 cup scallions
- Kosher salt
- ¼ cup cheddar cheese
- 2 eggs

Directions:
1. Heat the oven to 360 degrees F (182ºC). Then grease the baking dish with butter.
1. Put broccoli and 4 to 8 tablespoons water and place the bowl in the microwave for 3 minutes. Mix and again bake for 3 minutes.
2. Beat the eggs in a bowl. Pour all leftover items with broccoli.
3. Put all mixture in the baking dish. Bake for 30 minutes. Slice and serve.

Nutrition:
Calories: 196
Fat: 14g
Carbohydrate: 5 g
Protein: 12g
Fiber: 2 g

24. Low-Carb Broccoli Leek Soup

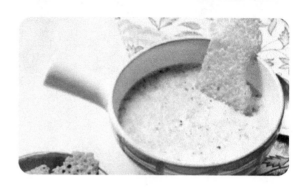

Preparation Time: 15 minutes
Cooking Time: 15 minutes
Servings: 2

Ingredients:
- ½ leek
- 3.5 oz (100 g) cream cheese
- 5.29 oz (150 g) broccoli
- ½ cup heavy cream
- 1 cup of water
- ¼ tablespoon black pepper
- ½ vegetable bouillon cube
- ¼ cup basil
- 1 teaspoon garlic
- Salt

Directions:
1. Put water into a pan and put broccoli chopped, leek chopped, and salt. Boil on high.
1. Simmer on low. Put the remaining items, simmer for 1 minute. Remove.
2. Blend the soup mixture into a blender. Serve.

Nutrition:
Calories: 545 kcal
Fat: 50 g
Carbohydrate: 10 g
Protein: 15g

25 Low-Carb Chicken Taco Soup

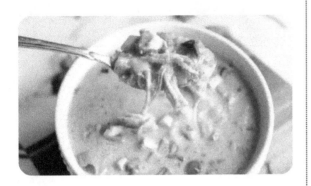

Preparation Time: 10 minutes
Cooking Time: 12 minutes
Servings: 2

Ingredients:
- 1 cup chicken broth
- ½ cup tomatoes
- ½ cup boneless chicken
- 4 green chilies
- ½ package cream cheese
- 1 tablespoon seasoning

Directions:
· Put chicken broth, boneless chicken, cheese, tomatoes, and green chilies in a pressure cooker.
· Cook for 10 minutes. Remove. Shred the chicken.
· Put shredded chicken in the soup and stir. Put Italian seasoning. Serve.

Nutrition:
Calories: 239
Fat: 12 g
Carbohydrate: 3 g
Protein: 26 g

26. Keto Chicken & Veggies Soup

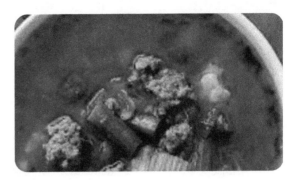

Preparation Time: 5 minutes
Cooking Time: 30 minutes
Servings: 2

Ingredients:
- ¼ tablespoon olive oil
- 1 cup chicken broth
- ½ onion
- ¼ tablespoon seasoning, Italian
- 2 bell peppers
- 1 spoon bay leaves
- ½ tablespoon garlic
- Sea salt
- ¼ cup green beans
- Black pepper
- ½ cup tomatoes
- 2 chicken breast pieces

Directions:
1. Massage the chicken with salt and pepper and grill for 10 minutes.
1. Put onions and bell pepper into heated oil and simmer for 5-6 minutes on low.
2. Add all leftover items and simmer for 15 minutes on low. Remove. Serve.

Nutrition:
Calories: 79
Fat: 2g
Carbohydrate: 11 g
Protein: 2g
Fiber: 3 g

27. Low-Carb Seafood Soup with Mayo

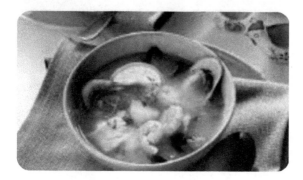

Preparation Time: 15 minutes
Cooking Time: 40 minutes
Servings: 2

Ingredients:

- ¼ tablespoon olive oil
- ½ chopped onion
- ¼ tablespoon garlic
- 2 cup fish broth
- 1 tomato
- thyme
- Salt
- Garlic mayo
- 3 oz. (85 grams) whitefish
- 1/3 cup olive oil
- 1/8 cup shrimps
- 1/3 garlic clove
- 1/8 cup mussels
- 1 egg,
- 1/8 cup scallops
- ½ tablespoon lemon juice
- 1/3 bay leaf
- Salt
- ½ lime

Directions:
1. Cook onions and garlic in heated olive oil. Put broth, bay leaf, tomatoes, and salt. After boiling, cover for 20 minutes on low flame.
1. Add all mixture and cook for 4 minutes.
2. Blend garlic mayo in the blender and put olive oil.
3. Put the mayo on the top middle and serve with thyme and lime.

Nutrition:
Calories: 592
Fat: 47g
Net **Carbohydrate:** 8 g
Protein: 27 g

28. Keto Tortilla Chips

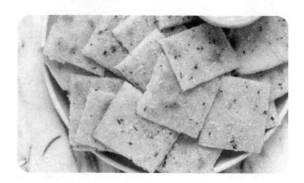

Preparation Time: 10 minutes
Cooking Time: 40 minutes
Servings: 2

Ingredients:

- ¼ cube of mozzarella cheese
- ¼ teaspoon cumin powder
- 0.7 oz (20 g) almond flour
- 1 teaspoon coriander
- 1 tablespoon cream cheese
- Chili powder
- 1 egg
- Salt

Directions:
1. Microwave the mozzarella cheese, cream cheese, and flour for 30 seconds. Stir and set for 30 seconds more.
1. Put spices and egg into the cheese mixture to make the dough.
2. Put the dough in two pieces of parchment paper in a large rectangular form.
3. Remove the parchment paper. Bake for 15 minutes to 400-degree F (204ºC).
4. Bake the other side of the dough in the same way.
5. Remove and cut into rectangular chips. Bake again for 2 minutes and serve.

Nutrition:
Calories: 198
Fat: 16 g
Carbohydrate: 4 g
Protein: 11 g

29. Chicken Zucchini Alfredo

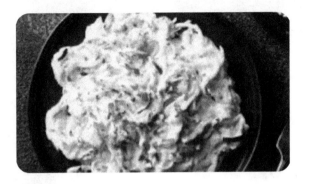

Preparation Time: 15 minutes
Cooking Time: 30 minutes
Servings: 2

Ingredients:
- 100 g (3.5 oz) chicken breast
- Basil
- 100 g (3.5 oz) zucchini
- 90 g (3.1 oz) cauliflower
- 40 g (1.41 oz) cream cheese
- Mayo
- Black pepper
- 1 teaspoon olive oil
- 1 teaspoon garlic

Directions:
1. Marinate chicken with basil, salt, and pepper. Grill the chicken and set aside.
1. Add oil, garlic, and zucchini
2. and cook for 8 to 10 minutes.
3. Put cream cheese in the zucchini with salt and pepper.
4. Let the cauliflower steam in the water. Mash the steamed cauliflower and put salt, pepper, and herbs.
5. Serve with mashed cauliflowers and enjoy an excellent lunch.

Nutrition:
Calories: 262.4
Fat: 9.8 g **Carbohydrate:** 13.7 g
Protein: 30.2g **Fiber:** 3.8 g

30. Low Carbs Chicken Cheese

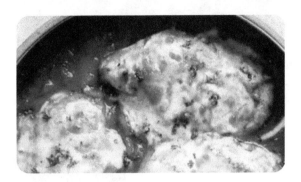

Preparation Time: 10 minutes
Cooking Time: 20 minutes
Servings: 2

Ingredients:
- 150 g (5.29 oz) chicken breast
- Salt
- ½ tablespoon Italian seasoning
- Pepper
- ½ teaspoon paprika
- ½ onion
- ¼ teaspoon onion powder
- 1 teaspoon garlic
- ½ tablespoon olive oil
- ½ fire-roasted pepper
- 425 g (14.1 oz) tomato
- Red pepper flakes
- ½ tablespoon parsley
- ¼ cup mozzarella cheese

Directions:
1. Marinate the chicken with salt, pepper, onion powder, and seasoning. Cook the chicken on low for 15 minutes.
1. Put the onion and all mixture except cheese and simmer for 7 minutes.
2. Put this sauce into a dish and place the cheese on the top of the chicken pieces. Warm-up for 1 to 2 minutes. Garnish with parsley and serve.

Nutrition:
Calories: 309
Fat: 9 g
Carbohydrate: 9 g
Protein: 37g
Fiber: 3 g

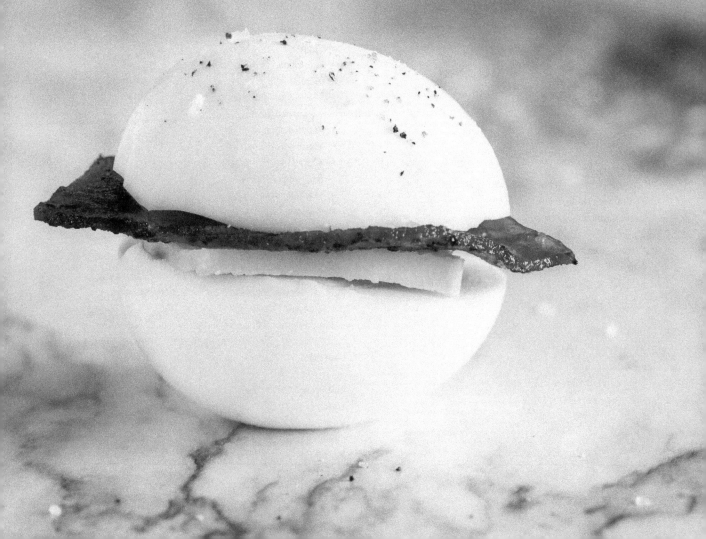

SNACK

31. Fried Green Beans Rosemary

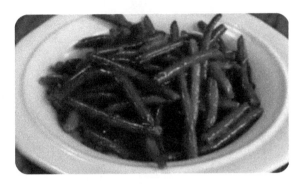

Preparation Time: 10 minutes
Cooking Time: 5 minutes
Servings: 2

Ingredients:
- green beans
- 3 tsp. minced garlic
- 2 tbsps. rosemary
- ½ tsp. salt
- 1 tbsp. butter

Directions:
Heat an Air Fryer to 390°F (199°C).
Put the chopped green beans then brush with butter.
Sprinkle salt, minced garlic, and rosemary over then cook for 5 minutes. Serve.

Nutrition:
Calories: 72
Fat: 6.3g
Protein: 0.7g
Carbohydrate: 4.5g

32. Crispy Broccoli Popcorn

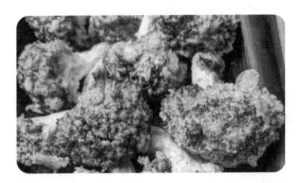

Preparation Time: 15 minutes
Cooking Time: 10 minutes
Servings: 4

Ingredients:
- 2 c. broccoli florets
- 2 c. coconut flour
- 4 egg yolks
- ½ tsp. salt
- ½ tsp. pepper
- ¼ c. butter

Directions:
Dissolve butter, then let it cool. Break the eggs in it.
Put coconut flour to the liquid, then put salt and pepper. Mix.
Heat an Air Fryer to 400°F (204°C).
Dip a broccoli floret in the coconut flour mixture, then place it in the Air Fryer.
Cook the broccoli florets 6 minutes. Serve.

Nutrition:
Calories: 202
Fat: 17.5g
Protein: 5.1g
Carbohydrate: 7.8g

33. Cheesy Cauliflower Croquettes

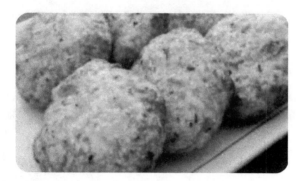

Preparation Time: 10 minutes
Cooking Time: 16 minutes
Servings: 4

Ingredients:
- 2 c. cauliflower florets
- 2 tsp. garlic
- ½ c. onion
- ¾ tsp. mustard
- ½ tsp. salt
- ½ tsp. pepper
- 2 tbsps. butter
- ¾ c. cheddar cheese

Directions:
· Microwave the butter. Let it cool.
· Process the cauliflower florets using a processor. Transfer to a bowl then put chopped onion and cheese.
· Put minced garlic, mustard, salt, and pepper, then pour melted butter over. Shape the cauliflower batter into medium balls.
· Heat an Air Fryer to 400°F (204°C)and cook for 14 minutes. Serve.

Nutrition:
Calories: 160
Fat: 13g
Protein: 6.8g
Carbohydrate: 5.1g

34. Spinach in Cheese Envelopes

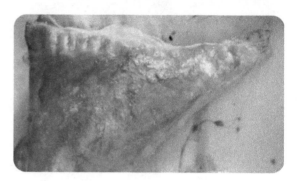

Preparation Time: 15 minutes
Cooking Time: 30 minutes
Servings: 8

Ingredients:
- 3 c. cream cheese
- 1½ c. coconut flour
- 3 egg yolks
- 2 eggs
- ½ c. cheddar cheese
- 2 c. steamed spinach
- ¼ tsp. salt
- ½ tsp. pepper
- ¼ c. onion

Directions:
1. Whisk cream cheese, put egg yolks. Stir in coconut flour until becoming a soft dough.
1. Put the dough on a flat surface then roll until thin. Cut the thin dough into 8 squares.
2. Beat the eggs, then place it in a bowl. Put salt, pepper, and grated cheese.
3. Put chopped spinach and onion to the egg batter.
4. Put spinach filling on a square dough then fold until becoming an envelope. Glue with water.
5. Heat an Air Fryer to 425°F (218°C). Cook for 12 minutes.
6. Remove and serve!

Nutrition:
Calories: 365
Fat: 34.6g
Protein: 10.4g
Carbohydrate: 4.4g

35. Cheesy Mushroom Slices

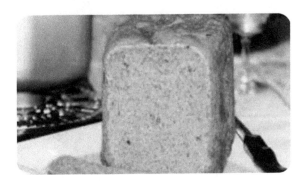

Preparation Time: 8-10 minutes
Cooking Time: 15 minutes
Servings: 8

Ingredients:
- 2 c. mushrooms
- 2 eggs
- ¾ c. almond flour
- ½ c. cheddar cheese
- 2 tbsps. butter
- ½ tsp. pepper
- ¼ tsp. salt

Directions:
1. Process chopped mushrooms in a food processor then add eggs, almond flour, and cheddar cheese.
1. Put salt and pepper then pour melted butter into the food processor. Transfer.
2. Heat an Air Fryer to 375°F (191°C).
3. Put the loaf pan on the Air Fryer's rack then cook for 15 minutes. Slice and serve.

Nutrition:
Calories: 365
Fat: 34.6g
Protein: 10.4g
Carbohydrate: 4.4g

36. Asparagus Fries

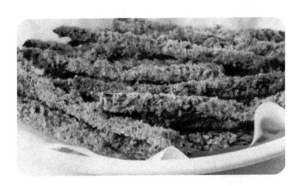

Preparation Time: 10 minutes
Cooking Time: 10 minutes
Servings: 4

Ingredients:
- 10 organic asparagus spears
- 1 tablespoon organic roasted red pepper
- ¼ almond flour
- ½ teaspoon garlic powder
- ½ teaspoon smoked paprika
- 2 tablespoons parsley
- ½ cup Parmesan cheese, full-fat
- 2 organic eggs
- 3 tablespoons mayonnaise, full-fat

Directions:
1. Heat the oven to 425 degrees F (218ºC).
1. Process cheese in a food processor, add garlic and parsley, and pulse for 1 minute.
2. Add almond flour, pulse for 30 seconds, transfer, and put paprika.
3. Whisk eggs into a shallow dish.
4. Dip asparagus spears into the egg batter, then coat with parmesan mixture and place it on a baking sheet. Bake in the oven for 10 minutes.
5. Put the mayonnaise in a bowl, add red pepper and whisk, then chill. Serve with prepared dip.

Nutrition:
Calories: 453 **Fat:** 33.4 g
Protein: 19.1 g Net **Carbohydrate:** 5.5 g

37. Kale Chips

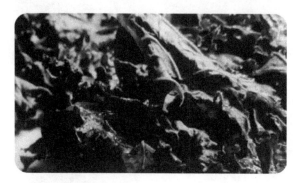

Preparation Time: 5 minutes
Cooking Time: 12 minutes
Servings: 4

Ingredients:

- 1 organic kale
- 1 tablespoon seasoned salt
- 2 tablespoons olive oil

Directions:

· Heat the oven to 350 degrees F (177ºC).
· Put kale leaves into a large plastic bag and add oil. Shake and then spread on a large baking sheet.
· Bake for 12 minutes. Serve with salt.

Nutrition:
Calories: 163
Fat: 10 g
Protein: 2 g
Carbohydrate: 14 g

38. Guacamole

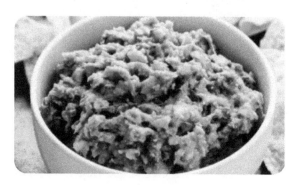

Preparation Time: 10 minutes
Cooking Time: 0 minutes
Servings: 4

Ingredients:

- 2 organic avocados pitted
- 1/3 organic red onion
- 1 organic jalapeño
- ½ teaspoon salt
- ½ teaspoon ground pepper
- 2 tablespoons tomato salsa
- 1 tablespoon lime juice
- ½ organic cilantro

Directions:
1. Slice the avocado flesh horizontally and vertically.
1. Mix in onion, jalapeno, and lime juice in a bowl.
2. Put salt and black pepper, add salsa, and mix. Add the cilantro and serve.
Nutrition:

Calories: 16.5
Fat: 1.4 g
Protein: 0.23 g
NetCarbohydrate: 0.5 g

39. Zucchini Noodles

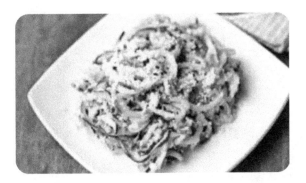

Preparation Time: 5 minutes
Cooking Time: 6 minutes
Servings: 2

Ingredients:
- 2 zucchinis, spiralized into noodles
- 2 tablespoons butter, unsalted
- 1 ½ tablespoon garlic
- ¾ cup Parmesan cheese
- ½ sea salt
- ¼ teaspoon ground black pepper
- ¼ teaspoon red chili flakes

Directions:
1. Sauté butter and garlic for 1 minute.
1. Put zucchini noodles, cook for 5 minutes, then put salt and black pepper.
2. Transfer then top with cheese and sprinkle with red chili flakes. Serve.

Nutrition:
Calories: 298
Fat: 26.1 g
Protein: 5 g
NetCarbohydrate: 2.3 g
Fiber: 0.1 g

40. Cauliflower Soufflé

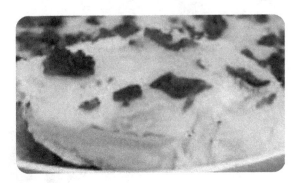

Preparation Time: 10 minutes
Cooking Time: 12 minutes
Servings: 6

Ingredients:
· 1 cauliflower, florets
· 2 eggs
· 2 tablespoons heavy cream
· 2 ounces cream Cheese
· ½ cup sour cream
· ½ cup Asiago cheese
· 1 cup cheddar cheese
· ¼ cup Chives
· 2 tablespoons butter, unsalted
· 6 bacon slices, sugar-free
· 1 cup of water

Directions:
Pulse eggs, heavy cream, sour cream, cream cheese, and cheeses in a food processor.
Put cauliflower florets, pulse for 2 seconds, then add butter and chives and pulse for another 2 seconds.
Put in water in a pot, and insert a trivet stand.
Put the cauliflower batter in a greased round casserole dish then put the dish on the trivet stand.
Cook for 12 minutes at high. Top with bacon, and serve.

Nutrition:
Calories: 342
Fat: 28; g
Protein: 17 g
Carbohydrate: 5 g

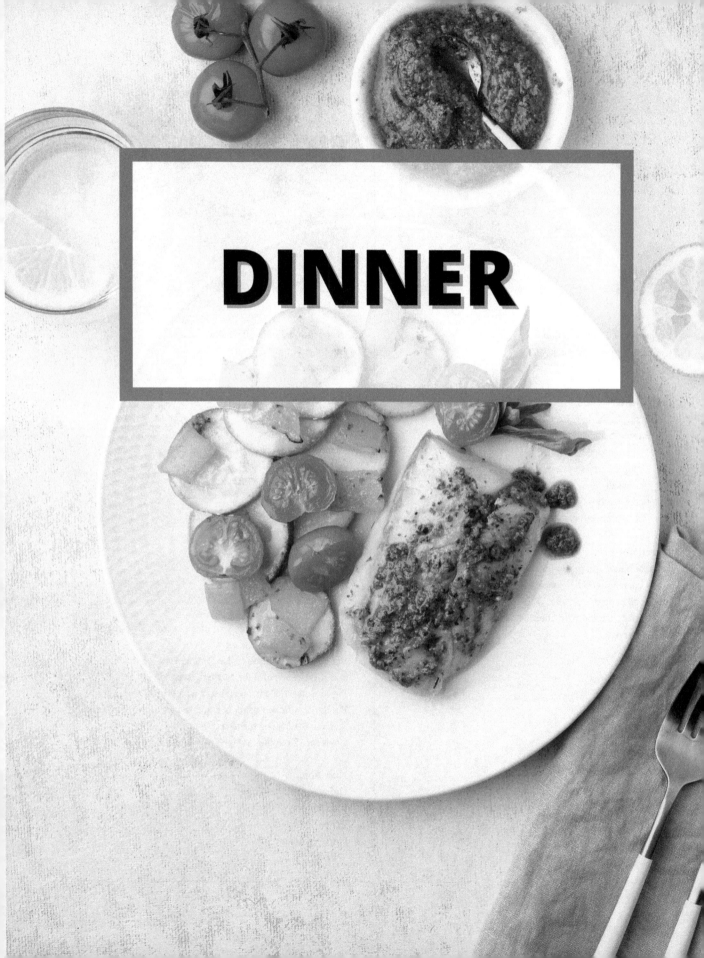

DINNER

41. Buttery Garlic Chicken

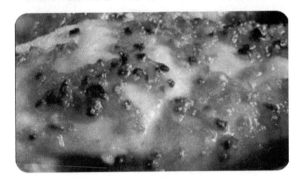

Preparation Time: 15 minutes
Cooking Time: 40 minutes
Servings: 2

Ingredients:
- 2 tablespoons ghee melted
- 2 boneless skinless chicken breasts
- 4 tablespoons butter
- 2 garlic cloves minced
- ¼ cup grated Parmesan cheese

Directions:
Heat the oven to 375 degrees F (191ºC), then choose a baking dish large enough to hold both chicken breasts and coat it with the ghee. Pat dry the chicken breasts and season with pink salt, pepper, and Italian seasoning. Place the chicken in the baking dish. Dissolve the butter in a skillet. Put the minced garlic and cook for 5 minutes, then remove the butter-garlic mixture from the heat and pour it over the chicken breasts. Roast the chicken in the oven for 30 to 35 minutes, until cooked through. Sprinkle some of the Parmesan cheese on top of each chicken breast. Let it rest in the baking dish for 5 minutes, then spoon the butter sauce over the chicken, and serve.

Nutrition:
Calories: 642
Carbohydrate: 2g
Protein: 57g
Fat: 45g

42. Creamy Slow Cooker Chicken

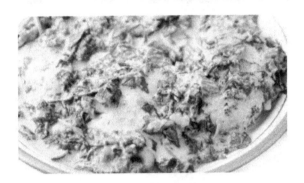

Preparation Time: 15 minutes
Cooking Time: 4 hours & 15 minutes
Servings: 2

Ingredients:
- 2 boneless skinless chicken breasts
- 1 cup Alfredo Sauce
- ¼ cup chopped sun-dried tomatoes
- ¼ cup Parmesan cheese, grated
- 2 cups fresh spinach

Directions:
Dissolve the ghee in a skillet, then put the chicken and cook, about 4 minutes on each side. With the crock insert in place, transfer the chicken to your slow cooker. Set your slow cooker to low. In a small bowl, mix the Alfredo sauce, sun-dried tomatoes, Parmesan cheese, salt, and pepper. Pour the sauce over the chicken. Cover and cook on low for 4 hours. Add the fresh spinach. Cover and cook for 5 minutes more, until the spinach is slightly wilted, and serve.

Nutrition:
Calories: 900
Carbohydrate: 9g
Protein: 70g
Fat: 66g

43. Braised Chicken Thighs with Kalamata Olives

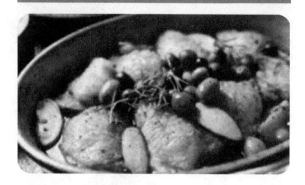

Preparation Time: 15 minutes
Cooking Time: 40 minutes
Servings: 2

Ingredients:
- 4 chicken thighs, skin on
- ½ cup chicken broth
- 1 lemon, ½ sliced and ½ juiced
- ½ cup pitted Kalamata olives
- 2 tablespoons butter

Directions:
Heat the oven to 375 degrees F (191ºC), then dry chicken, and season to taste. In a medium oven-safe skillet or high-sided baking dish over medium-high heat, melt butter. When the butter has melted and is hot, add the chicken thighs, skin-side down, and leave them for about 8 minutes, or until the skin is brown and crispy. Turn over the chicken and cook for 2 minutes on the second side. Around the chicken thighs, pour in the chicken broth, and add the lemon slices, lemon juice, and olives. Bake in the oven for about 30 minutes, until the chicken is cooked through. Add the butter to the broth mixture. Divide the chicken and olives between two plates and serve.

Nutrition:
Calories: 567
Carbohydrate: 4g
Protein: 33g
Fat: 47g

44. Baked Garlic and Paprika Chicken Legs

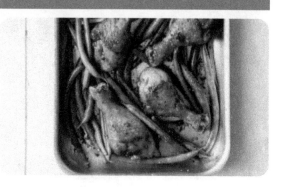

Preparation Time: 15 minutes
Cooking Time: 60 minutes
Servings: 2

Ingredients:
- 1 lb. chicken drumsticks, skin on
- 2 tablespoons paprika
- 2 garlic cloves minced
- ½ pound fresh green beans
- 1 tablespoon olive oil

Directions:
Set oven to 350˚F (177ºC). Combine all the ingredients in a large bowl, toss to combine, and transfer to a baking dish. Bake for 60 minutes until crisp and thoroughly cooked.

Nutrition:
Calories: 700
Carbohydrate: 10g
Protein: 63g
Fat: 45g

45. Chicken Curry with Masala

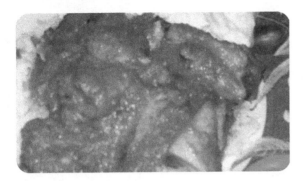

Preparation Time: 15 minutes
Cooking Time: 30 minutes
Servings: 4

Ingredients:
- 2 tbsp.of oil
- 2 tbsp.of minced jalapeño
- 1 ½ pound (680 g) of diced boneless skinless chicken thighs
- 1 tsp. of garam masala
- ¼ cup of chopped cilantro
- 2 tbsp.of diced ginger
- 1 cup of chopped tomatoes
- 2 tsp. of turmeric
- 1 tsp. of cayenne
- 2 tbsp. of lemon juice
- 1 tsp. of garam masala

Directions:
Heat your Air Fryer to a temperature of about 400° F (204°C). Grease the Air Fryer pan with the cooking spray. Add the jalapenos and the ginger. Add in the chicken and the tomatoes and stir. Add the spices and 1 tbsp. of oil and 1 tbsp.of water. Place the pan in Air Fryer and set the temperature to 365° F (185°C). Now, set the timer to 30 minutes. When the timer beeps, turn off your Air Fryer. Serve and enjoy your lunch!

Nutrition:
Calories: 254
Carbohydrate: 9g
Protein: 27.8g
Fat: 14g

46.1. Chicken Quesadilla

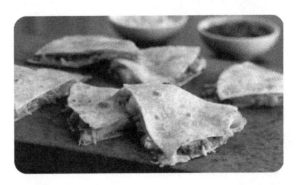

Preparation Time: 15 minutes
Cooking Time: 5 minutes
Servings: 2

Ingredients:
- 1 tablespoon olive oil
- 2 low-carbohydrate tortillas
- ½ cup shredded Mexican blend cheese
- 2 ounces (56 g) shredded chicken
- 2 tablespoons sour cream

Directions:
Heat the olive oil in a large skillet, then put a tortilla, then top with ¼ cup of cheese, the chicken, the Tajin seasoning, and the remaining ¼ cup of cheese. Top with the second tortilla. Once the bottom tortilla gets golden, and the cheese begins to melt, after about 2 minutes, flip the quesadilla over. The second side will cook faster, about 1 minute. Once the second tortilla is crispy and golden, transfer the quesadilla to a cutting board and let sit for 2 minutes. Cut the quesadilla into 4 wedges using a pizza cutter or chef's knife. Transfer half the quesadilla to each of two plates. Put 1 tablespoon of sour cream and serve hot.

Nutrition:
Calories: 414
Carbohydrate: 24g
Protein: 26g
Fat: 28g

47. Slow Cooker Barbecue Ribs

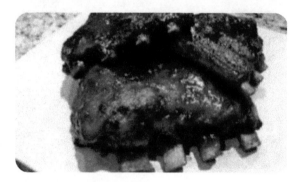

Preparation Time: 15 minutes
Cooking Time: 4 hours
Servings: 2

Ingredients:
- 1 lb. (453 g) pork ribs
- Pink salt
- Freshly ground black pepper
- 1.25 oz. (35.4 g) package dry rib-seasoning rub
- ½ cup sugar-free barbecue sauce

Directions:
With the crock insert in place, preheat your slow cooker to high. Generously season the pork ribs with pink salt, pepper, and dry rib-seasoning rub. Stand the ribs up along the walls of the slow-cooker insert, with the bonier side facing inward. Pour the barbecue sauce on both sides of the ribs, using just enough to coat. Cover, cook for 4 hours, and serve.

Nutrition:
Calories: 956
Carbohydrate: 5g
Protein: 68g
Fat: 72g

48. Barbacoa Beef Roast

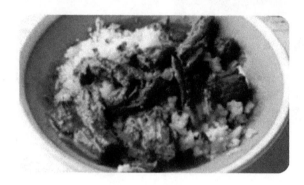

Preparation Time: 15 minutes
Cooking Time: 8 hours
Servings: 4

Ingredients:
- 1 lb. (453 g) beef chuck roast
- 4 chipotle peppers in adobo sauce
- 6 oz. (170 g) can green jalapeño chiles
- 2 tablespoons apple cider vinegar
- ½ cup beef broth

Directions:
With the crock insert in place, preheat your slow cooker to low. Massage the beef chuck roast on both sides with pink salt and pepper. Put the roast in the slow cooker. Pulse the chipotle peppers and their adobo sauce, jalapeños, and apple cider vinegar in a blender. Add the beef broth and pulse a few more times. Pour the chili mixture over the top of the roast. Cover and cook on low for 8 hours, then shred the meat. Serve hot.
Nutrition:
Calories: 723
Carbohydrate: 7g
Protein: 66g
Fat: 46g

49. Beef & Broccoli Roast

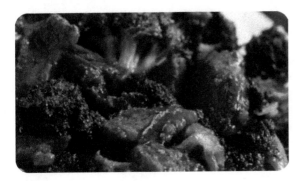

Preparation Time: 15 minutes
Cooking Time: 4 hours & 30 minutes
Servings: 2

Ingredients:
- 1 lb. (453 g) beef chuck roast
- ½ cup beef broth
- ¼ cup soy sauce
- 1 teaspoon toasted sesame oil
- 1 (16-ounce/454 g) bag frozen broccoli

Directions:
With the crock insert in place, preheat your slow cooker to low. On a cutting board, season the chuck roast with pink salt and pepper, and slice the roast thin. Put the sliced beef in your slow cooker. Combine sesame oil and beef broth in a small bowl then pour over the beef. Cover and cook on low for 4 hours. Add the frozen broccoli and cook for 30 minutes more. If you need more liquid, add additional beef broth. Serve hot.

Nutrition:
Calories: 803
Carbohydrate: 18g
Protein: 74g
Fat: 49g

50. Cauliflower and Pumpkin Casserole

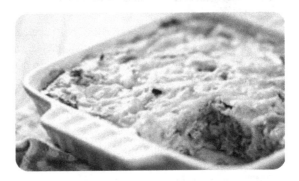

Preparation Time: 15 minutes
Cooking Time: 1 hour & 30 minutes
Servings: 4

Ingredients:
- 2 tbsp. olive oil
- ¼ medium yellow onion, minced
- 6 cups chopped forage kale into small pieces (about 140 g /5 oz)
- 1 little clove garlic, minced
- Salt and freshly ground black pepper
- ½ cup low sodium chicken broth
- 2 cups of 1.5 cm diced pumpkin (about 230 g/8.11 oz)
- 2 cups of 1.5 cm diced zucchini (about 230 g/8.11 oz)
- 2 tbsp.mayonnaise
- 3 cups frozen, thawed brown rice
- 1 cup grated Swiss cheese
- 1/3 cup grated Parmesan
- 1 cup panko flour
- 1 large beaten egg
- Cooking spray

Directions:
1. Preheat oven to 200 ° C (392ºF). Heat the oil in a large non-stick skillet over medium heat. Add onions and cook, occasionally stirring, until browned and tender (about 5 minutes). Add the cabbage, garlic, ½ teaspoon salt, and ½ teaspoon pepper and cook until the cabbage is light (about 2 minutes).

1. Put the stock and cook for 5 minutes, then put the squash, zucchini, and ½ teaspoon Salt and mix well. Continuously cooking for 8 minutes. Remove from heat and add mayonnaise.

2. In a bowl, combine cooked vegetables, brown rice, cheese, ½ cup flour, and large egg and mix well. Spray a 2-liter casserole with cooking spray. Put the mixture to the pan and cover with the remaining flour, ¼ teaspoon salt, and a few pinches of pepper. Bake until the squash and zucchini are tender and the top golden and crispy (about 35 minutes). Serve hot.

Advanced Preparation Tip: Freeze the casserole for up to 2 weeks. Cover with aluminum foil and heat at 180°C (356ºF) until warm (35 to 45 minutes).

Nutrition:

Calories: 83

Carbohydrate: 11g

Fat: 3g

Protein: 5g

51. Portobello Pizza

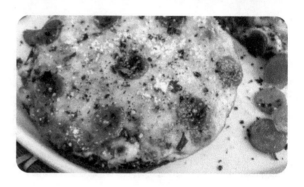

Preparation Time: 15 minutes

Cooking Time: 6 minutes

Servings: 1

Ingredients:

- 1½ oz. (42.5 g) Monterey jack
- 9 spinach leaves
- 3 Portobello mushrooms
- 1½ oz. cheddar cheese
- Olive oil
- 1½ oz. mozzarella
- 12 pepperoni slices
- 3 tomato slices
- 3 tsp. pizza seasoning

Directions:

1. Through cleaning them and cutting the gills and the stalks, dress the Portobello mushrooms.

2. Sprinkle with the seasoning of olive oil and bread, and add the other ingredients, except the pepperoni. Cook 6 minutes at 450°F (232ºC). Add the slices of pepperoni and grill until crumbly.

Nutrition:

Calories: 250

Carbohydrate: 23g

Fat: 13g

Protein: 18g

52. Turkey Mozzarella Burgers

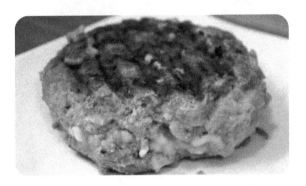

Preparation Time: 10 minutes
Cooking Time: 6 minutes
Servings: 2

Ingredients:

- 8 ounces (227 g) ground turkey
- 1 ounce (28 g) mozzarella cheese, cubed
- Salt and black pepper, to taste
- 1 tbsp. butter

Directions:

1. In a bowl, add all the turkey, salt and black pepper and mix until well combined. Make 2 equal sized patties from the mixture.
2. Place mozzarella cubes inside each patty and cover with the meat. In a frying pan, melt butter over medium heat and cook patties for about 2-3 minutes per side. Serve hot.

Nutrition:
Calories: 312
Carbohydrate: 0.5g
Fat: 20g
Protein: 35g

53. Grilled Chicken Salad with Oranges

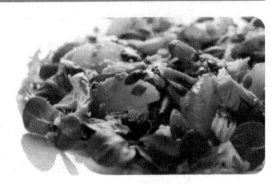

Preparation Time: 15 minutes
Cooking Time: 15 minutes
Servings: 4

Ingredients:

- 75 ml (1/3 cup) orange juice
- 30 ml (2 tablespoons) lemon juice
- 45 ml (3 tablespoons) of extra virgin olive oil
- 15 ml (1 tablespoon) Dijon mustard
- 2 cloves of garlic, chopped
- 1 ml (¼ teaspoon) Salt
- Freshly ground pepper
- 1 lb. (453 g) skinless chicken breast, trimmed
- 25 g (¼ cup/0.8 oz) pistachio or flaked almonds, toasted
- 600 g (8c/5 oz) of mesclun, rinsed and dried
- 75 g (½ cup/2.6 oz) minced red onion
- 2 medium oranges, peeled, quartered and sliced

Directions:

1. Place the orange juice, lemon juice, oil, mustard, garlic, salt, and pepper in a small bowl or jar with an airtight lid; whip or shake to mix. Reserve 75 milliliters of this salad vinaigrette and 45 milliliters for basting.
2. Place the rest of the vinaigrette in a shallow glass dish or resealable plastic bag. Add the chicken and turn it over to coat. Cover or close and marinate in the refrigerator for at least 20 minutes or up to two hours.
3. Preheat the barbecue over medium heat. Lightly oil the grill by rubbing it with a crumpled paper towel soaked in oil.

Grill the chicken 10 to 15 centimeters (four to six inches) from the heat source, basting the cooked sides with the basting vinaigrette until it is no longer pink in the center, and Instant-read thermometer inserted in the thickest part records 75 ° C (170 ° F), four to six minutes on each side. Transfer then let it rest for five minutes.

4.Meanwhile, grill almonds in a small, dry pan on medium-low heat, stirring constantly, until lightly browned, about two to three minutes. Transfer them to a bowl and let them cool.

5.Place the salad and onion mixture in a large bowl then mix with the vinaigrette reserved for the salad. Slice chicken and spread on salads. Sprinkle orange slices on top and sprinkle with pistachios.

Nutrition:
Calories: 290
Carbohydrate: 21g
Fat: 14g
Protein: 25g

54.Classic Chicken Salad

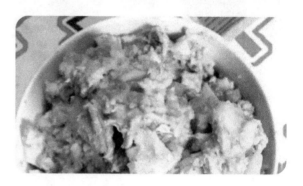

Preparation Time: 15 minutes
Cooking Time: 0 minutes
Servings: 4

Ingredients:
- 1 medium shallot, thinly sliced
- 1 tablespoon Dijon mustard
- 1 tablespoon fresh oregano, chopped
- 1/2 cup mayonnaise
- 2 cups boneless rotisserie chicken, shredded
- 2 avocados, pitted, peeled and diced
- Salt and black pepper, to taste
- 3 hard-boiled eggs, cut into quarters

Directions:
1. Toss the chicken with the avocado, shallots, and oregano.
2. Add in the mayonnaise, mustard, salt and black pepper; stir to combine.

Nutrition:
Calories: 290
Carbohydrate: 19g
Fat: 13g
Protein: 27g

55. Chicken Fillet with Brussel Sprouts

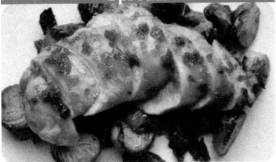

Preparation Time: 15 minutes
Cooking Time: 10 minutes
Servings: 4
Ingredients:

- 3/4 pound (340 g) chicken breasts, chopped into bite-sized pieces
- 1/2 teaspoon ancho chile powder
- 1/2 teaspoon whole black peppercorns
- 1/2 cup onions, chopped
- 1 cup vegetable broth
- 2 tablespoons olive oil
- 1 ½ pounds (680 g) Brussels sprouts, trimmed and cut into halves
- 1/4 teaspoon garlic salt
- 1 clove garlic, minced
- 2 tablespoons port wine

Directions:

1. Heat 1 tablespoon of the oil in a frying pan over medium-high heat. Sauté the Brussels sprouts for about 3 minutes or until golden on all sides. Salt to taste and reserve.

2. Heat the remaining tablespoon of olive oil. Cook the garlic and chicken for about 3 minutes. Add in the onions, vegetable broth, wine, ancho chile powder, and black peppercorns; bring to a boil.

3. Then, reduce the temperature to simmer and continue to cook for 4 to 5 minutes longer. Add the reserved Brussels sprouts back to the frying pan.

Nutrition:
Calories: 38
Carbohydrate: 8g
Fat: 3g
Protein: 3g

56. Italian Keto Casserole

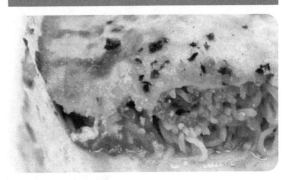

Preparation Time: 15 minutes
Cooking Time: 1 hour
Servings: 4
Ingredients:

- 200 g (9 oz) Shirataki noodles
- 2 tbsp. olive oil
- 1 small onion, diced
- 2 garlic cloves, finely chopped
- 1 tsp. dried marjoram
- 450 g (16 oz) ground beef
- 1 tsp. Salt
- ½ tsp. ground pepper
- 2 chopped tomatoes
- 1 cup of fat cream
- 340 g (12 oz) ricotta cheese
- ⅓ cup grated parmesan
- 1 egg
- ¼ cup parsley, roughly chopped

Directions:

1. Preheat the oven to 190ºC (374ºF).

2. Prepare the shirataki noodles as indicated on the packaging, strain well, and set aside.

3. Cook oil, onion, garlic, marjoram, and fry for 2-3 minutes, until the onion is soft.

4. Add ground beef, salt and pepper, and simmer, stirring, while the mixture is browned.

5. Add tomatoes and fat cream, and cook for 5 minutes.

6. Remove from heat and mix with noodles. Transfer the mixture to a baking dish.

7. Mix ricotta, parmesan, egg, and parsley. Spoon over the casserole.

8. Bake about 35-45 minutes until golden brown.

Nutrition:
Calories: 275
Carbohydrate: 0g
Fat: 10g

57. Salmon Keto Cutlets

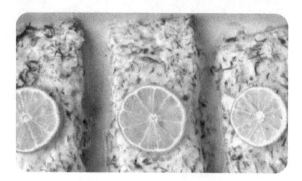

Preparation Time: 15 minutes
Cooking Time: 10 minutes
Servings: 4

Ingredients:
- 450 g (or 1 lb) canned salmon
- ½ cup almond flour
- ¼ cup shallots, finely chopped
- 2 tbsp. parsley, finely chopped
- 1 tbsp.dried chopped onions
- 2 large eggs
- Zest of 1 lemon
- 1 clove garlic, finely chopped
- ½ tsp. Salt
- ½ tsp. ground white pepper
- 3 tbsp. olive oil

Directions:
1. Put all the mixture except the oil in a large bowl and mix well.
1. Form 8, identical cutlets.
2. Fry salmon cutlets in portions, adding more oil as needed, for 2-3 minutes on each side.
3. Serve the cutlets warm or cold with lemon wedges and low carbohydrate mayonnaise.

Nutrition:
Calories: 300
Carbohydrate: 0g
Fat: 19g
Protein: 35g

58. Baked Cauliflower

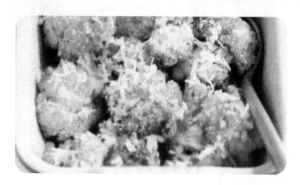

Preparation Time: 15 minutes
Cooking Time: 60 minutes
Servings: 2
Ingredients:
- 1 medium cauliflower
- 113 g (4 oz) of salted butter
- ⅓ cup finely grated parmesan
- 3 tbsp. Dijon mustard
- 2 minced garlic cloves
- Zest of 1 lemon
- ½ tsp. Salt
- ½ tsp. ground pepper
- 28 g (1 oz) fresh Parmesan
- 1 tbsp. finely chopped parsley

Directions:
· Preheat the oven to 190ºC (374ºF).
· Put the cauliflower in a small baking dish.
· Put the remaining ingredients in a small saucepan, except for fresh parmesan and parsley, and put on low heat until they melt. Whip together.
· Lubricate cauliflower ⅓ of the oil mixture.
· Bake for 20 minutes, then remove from the oven and pour another quarter of the oil mixture.
· Bake for another 20 minutes and pour over the remaining oil mixture.
· Cook for another 20-30 minutes until the core is soft.
· Put on a plate, sprinkle a drop of oil from the mold, grate fresh parmesan and sprinkle with parsley.

Nutrition:
Calories: 1
Carbohydrate: 4g
Fat: 11g
Protein: 1g

59. Risotto with Mushrooms

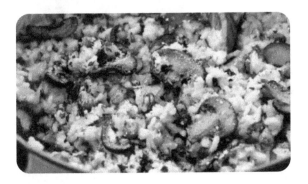

Preparation Time: 15 minutes
Cooking Time: 25 minutes
Servings: 2

Ingredients:
- 2 tbsp. olive oil
- 2 minced garlic cloves
- 1 small onion, finely diced
- 1 tsp. salt
- ½ tsp. ground white pepper
- 200 g (7 oz) chopped mushrooms
- ¼ cup chopped oregano leaves
- 255 g (9 oz) cauliflower "rice"
- ¼ cup vegetable broth
- 2 tbsp.butter
- ⅓ cup grated parmesan

Directions:
Sauté oil, garlic, onions, salt, and pepper, and sauté for 5-7 minutes until the onions become transparent.
Add mushrooms and oregano, and cook for 5 minutes.
Add cauliflower rice and vegetable broth, then reduce heat to medium. Cook the risotto, frequently stirring, for 10-15 minutes, until the cauliflower is soft.
Remove from heat, and mix with butter and parmesan.
Try and add more seasoning if you want.

Nutrition:
Calories: 206
Carbohydrate: 31g
Fat: 7g
Protein: 4g

60. Low Carb Green Bean Casserole

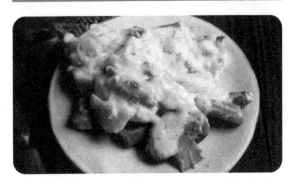

Preparation Time: 15 minutes
Cooking Time: 60 minutes
Servings: 4
Ingredients:
- 2 tbsp.butter
- 1 small chopped onion
- 2 minced garlic cloves
- 226.8 g (8 oz) chopped mushrooms
- ½ tsp. salt
- ½ tsp. ground pepper
- ½ cup chicken stock
- ½ cup of fat cream
- ½ tsp. xanthan gum
- 453.59 g (16 oz) green beans (with cut ends)
- 56.7 g (2 oz) crushed cracklings

Directions:
1.Preheat the oven to 190ºC (374ºF).
2.Add oil, onion, and garlic to a non-stick pan over high heat. Fry until onion is transparent.
3.Add mushrooms, salt, and pepper. Cook for 7 minutes until the mushrooms are tender.
· Add chicken stock and cream, and bring to a boil. Sprinkle with xanthan gum, mix and cook for 5 minutes.
4.Add the string beans to the creamy mixture and pour it into the baking dish.
5.Cover with foil and bake for 20 minutes.
6.Remove the foil, sprinkle with greaves and bake for another 10-15 minutes.

Nutrition:
Calories: 244
Carbohydrate: 6g
Fat: 18g
Protein: 8g

DESSERT

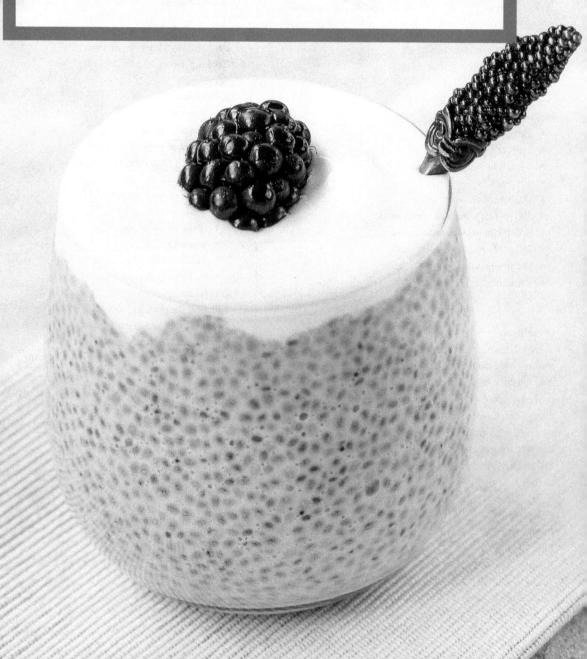

61. Keto and Dairy-Free Vanilla Custard

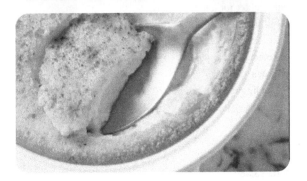

Preparation Time: 11 minutes
Cooking Time: 5 minutes
Servings: 4

Ingredients:
- 6 egg yolks
- ½ cup unsweetened almond milk
- 1 tsp. vanilla extract
- ¼ cup melted coconut oil

Directions:
1. Mix egg yolks, almond milk, vanilla in a metal bowl.
1. Gradually stir in the melted coconut oil.
2. Boil water in a saucepan, place the mixing bowl over the saucepan.
3. Whisk the mixture constantly and vigorously until thickened for about 5 minutes.
4. Remover from the saucepan, serve hot or chill in the fridge.

Nutrition:
Calories: 215.38
Fat: 21g
Carbohydrate: 1g
Protein: 4g

62. Keto Triple Chocolate Mug Cake

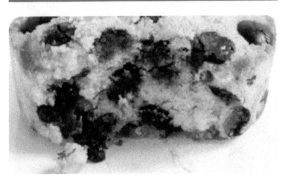

Preparation Time: 3 minutes
Cooking Time: 1 minute
Servings: 3

Ingredients:
- 1 ½ tbsp. coconut flour
- ½ tsp. baking powder
- 2 tbsp. cacao powder
- 2 tbsp. powdered sweetener
- 1 medium egg
- 5 tbsp. double/heavy cream
- 2 tbsp. sugar-free chocolate chips
- ¼ tsp. vanilla extract optional

Directions:
1. Mix all dry mixture- coconut flour, baking powder, cacao powder, and a bowl.
1. Whisk together the egg, cream, and vanilla extract, pour the mixture in the dry ingredients.
2. Add the chocolate chips in the mixture and let the batter rest for a minute.
3. Grease the ramekins with the melted butter, pour the batter in the ramekins.
4. Place in the microwave and microwave for 1 ½ minute until cooked through.

Nutrition:
Calories: 250
Carbohydrate: 9.7g
Protein: 6g
Fat: 22g

63. Keto Cheesecake Stuffed Brownies

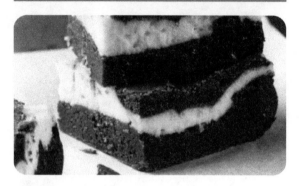

Preparation Time: 11 minutes
Cooking Time: 30 minutes
Servings: 16

Ingredients:
For the Filling:
- 8 oz (225g) cream cheese
- ¼ cup sweetener
- 1 large egg
- For the Brownie:
- 3 oz (85g) low carb milk chocolate
- 5 tbsp. butter
- 3 large eggs
- ½ cup sweetener
- ¼ cup cocoa powder
- ½ cup almond flour

Directions:
·1.Heat-up oven to 350 °F (177ºC), line a brownie pan with parchment.
2.In a mixing bowl, whisk together cream cheese, egg, and sweetener until smooth, set aside.
3.Place chocolate and butter in a microwave-safe bowl and microwave at 30 seconds interval.
4.Whisk frequently until smooth, allow to cool for a few minutes.
5.Whisk together the remaining eggs and sweetener until fluffy.

Mix in the almond flour plus cocoa powder until soft peaks form.
6.Mix in the chocolate and butter mixture and beat with a hand mixer for a few seconds.
7.Fill the prepared pan with ¾ of the batter, then top with the cream cheese and the brownie batter. Bake the cheesecake brownie until mostly set for about 25-30 minutes.
8.The jiggling parts of the cake will firm when you remove it from the oven.

Nutrition:
Calories: 143.94
Fat: 13.48g
Carbohydrate: 1.9g
Protein: 3.87g

64. Keto Raspberry Ice Cream

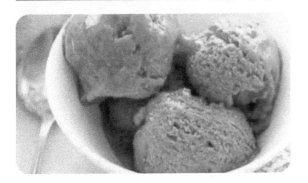

Preparation Time: 45 minutes
Cooking Time: 0 minutes
Servings: 8

Ingredients:
- 2 cups heavy whipping cream
- 1 cup raspberries
- ½ cup powdered erythritol
- 1 pasteurized egg yolk

Directions:
1. Process all the ice cream ingredients in a food processor.
2. Add blended mixture into the ice cream maker.
3. Turn on the ice cream machine and churn according to the manufacturer's directions.

Nutrition:
Calories: 120
Fat: 23g
Carbohydrate: 4g
Protein: 0g

65. Chocolate Macadamia Nut Fat Bombs

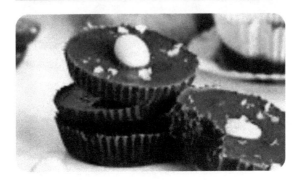

Preparation Time: 11 minutes
Cooking Time: 30 minutes
Servings: 4

Ingredients:
- 1⅓ oz (38g) sugar-free dark chocolate
- 1 tbsp. coconut oil
- coarse salt or sea salt
- 1½ oz (42g) raw macadamia nuts halves

Directions:
1. Put three macadamia nut halves in each of 8 wells of the mini muffin pan.
1. Microwave the chocolate chips for about a few seconds.
2. Whisk until smooth, add coconut oil and salt, mix until well combined.
3. Fill the mini muffin pan with the chocolate mixture to cover the nuts completely.
4. Refrigerate the muffin pan until chilled and firm for about 30 minutes.

Nutrition:
Calories: 153
Fat: 1g
Carbohydrate: 2g
Protein: 4g

66. Keto Peanut Butter Chocolate Bars

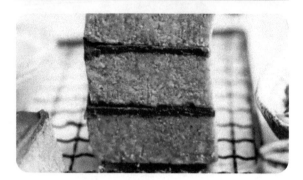

Preparation Time: 11 minutes
Cooking Time: 10 minutes
Servings: 8

Ingredients:
For the Bars:
- 3/4 cup (84 g) Superfine Almond Flour
- 2 oz (56.7 g) Butter
- ¼ cup (45.5 g) Swerve, Icing sugar style
- ½ cup Peanut Butter
- 1 tsp. Vanilla extract

For the Topping:
- ½ cup (90 g) Sugar-Free Chocolate Chips

Directions:
1.Combine all the ingredients for the bars and spread into a small 6-inch pan.
2.Microwave the chocolate in the microwave oven for 30 seconds and whisk until smooth.
3.Pour the melted chocolate in over the bars ingredients.
4.Refrigerate for at least an hour or two until the bars firmed. Keep in an airtight container.

Nutrition:
Calories: 246
Fat: 23g
Carbohydrate: 7g
Protein: 7g

67. Salted Toffee Nut Cups

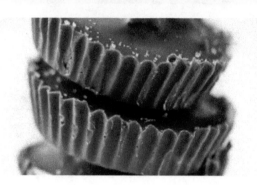

Preparation Time: 11 minutes
Cooking Time: 10 minutes
Servings: 5

Ingredients:
- 5 oz (141g) low-carb milk chocolate
- 3 tbsp.+ 2 tbsp.sweetener
- 3 tbsp.cold butter
- ½ oz (14g) raw walnuts, chopped
- Sea salt to taste

Directions:
1. Microwave the chocolate in 45 seconds intervals and continue whisk until chocolate melted.
1. Line the cupcake pan with 5 paper liners and add chocolate to the bottom of the cupcake.
2. Spread the chocolate to coat the bottom of the cupcake evenly, freeze to harden.
3. In a heat-proof bowl, heat the cold butter and sweetener on power 8 for three minutes.
4. Stir the butter every 20 seconds to prevent the burning.
5. Mix in the 2 tbsp. of sweetener and whisk to thicken. Fold in the walnuts.
6. Fill the chocolate cups with the toffee mixture quickly.
7. Top the cupcakes with the remaining chocolate and refrigerate to firm for 20-30 minutes.
8. Remove from the cups and sprinkle with sea salt!

Nutrition:
Calories: 194
Fat: 18g
Carbohydrate: 2g
Protein: 2.5g

68. Crisp Meringue Cookies

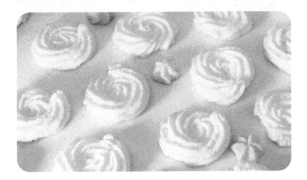

Preparation Time: 10 minutes
Cooking Time: 40 minutes
Servings: 8

Ingredients:
- 4 large egg whites
- ¼ tsp. cream of tartar
- ½ tsp. almond extract
- 6 tbsp.Swerve Confectioners
- Pinch of salt

Directions:
1. Preheat oven to 210 °F (100 °C).
2. Whip egg whites, cream of tartar in a mixing bowl on medium speed until foamy.
3. While whipping, gradually add the swerve confectioners ¼ tsp. at a time.
4. When all the swerve added ultimately, then turn the mixer up to high speed and whip.
5. Add in the almond extract and whip until very stiff.
6. Pour the batter in a piping bag with a French star tip and pipe the batter onto the lined baking
7. Sheet. Bake the meringue for 40 minutes.
8. Serve immediately, enjoy!

Nutrition:
Calories: 4
Fat: 0.01g
Carbohydrate: 0.09g
Protein: 0.08g

69. Instant Pot Matcha Cheesecake

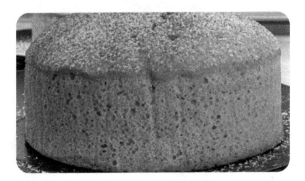

Preparation Time: 11 minutes
Cooking Time: 55 minutes
Servings: 6
Ingredients:
Cheesecake:
- 16 oz (450g) cream cheese, room temperature
- ½ cup sweetener
- 2 tsp. coconut flour
- ½ tsp. vanilla extract
- 2 tbsp. heavy whipping cream
- 1 tbsp. matcha powder
- 2 large eggs, room temperature

Directions:
· In a mixing bowl, combine cream cheese, Swerve, coconut flour, vanilla extract, whipping cream, and matcha powder until well combined. Stir in the eggs one at a time.
· Add the cheesecake batter into the prepared springform pan.
· Pour 1 ½ cups of water into the bottom of the Instant Pot. Put the trivet in the instant pot.
· Place the springform on the top of the trivet, sealing, and securing the instant pot's lid.
· Set the instant pot on high pressure, set the timing for 35 minutes.
· Once the cooking time is up, release the pressure naturally.
· Transfer the cheesecake on a cooling rack and allow it to cool the cake for 30 minutes.
· Top with your favorite toppings, enjoy!
Nutrition:
Calories: 350
Fat: 33.2g
Carbohydrate: 5.8g
Protein: 8.4g

70. Matcha Skillet Soufflé

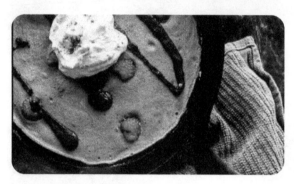

Preparation Time: 5 minutes
Cooking Time: 5 minutes
Servings: 1

Ingredients:

- 3 large eggs
- 2 tbsp.sweetener
- 1 tsp. vanilla extract
- 1 tbsp. matcha powder
- 1 tbsp. butter
- 7 whole raspberries
- 1 tbsp.coconut oil
- 1 tbsp. unsweetened cocoa powder
- ¼ cup whipped cream

Directions:

1. Broil, then heat-up a heavy-bottom pan over medium heat.

1. Whip the egg whites with one tablespoon of Swerve confectioners. Once the peaks form to add in the matcha powder, whisk again.

2. With a fork, break up the yolks. Mix in the vanilla, then add a little amount of the whipped whites. Carefully fold the remaining of the whites into the yolk mixture.

3. Dissolve the butter in a pan, put the soufflé mixture to the pan. Reduce the heat to low and top with raspberries. Cook until the eggs double in size and set.

4. Transfer the pan to the oven and keep an eye on it. Cook until golden browned.

5. Melt the coconut oil and combine with cocoa powder and the remaining Swerve.

6. Drizzle the chocolate mixture across the top.

Nutrition:
Calories 578
Fat: 50.91g
Carbohydrate: 5.06g
Protein: 20.95g

30 Days Meal Plan

Day 1. Mushroom Omelet - Turkey Meatballs - Cauliflower Soufflé - Beef & Broccoli Roast. - Matcha Skillet Soufflé

Day 2. Keto Waffles and Blueberries - Cauliflower Leek Soup - Fried Green Beans Rosemary - Portobello Pizza Keto and Dairy-Free Vanilla Custard

Day 3. Cream cheese eggs - Zucchini Sushi - Crispy Broccoli Popcorn - Braised Chicken Thighs with Kalamata Olives -
   Keto Cheesecake Stuffed Brownies

Day 4. Creamy Basil Baked Sausage - Chicken Tacos - Spinach in Cheese Envelopes - Baked Garlic and Paprika Chicken Legs - Keto Raspberry Ice Cream

Day 5. Almond Coconut Egg Wraps - California Burger Bowls - Cheesy Mushroom Slices - Cauliflower and Pumpkin Casserole - Chocolate Macadamia Nut Fat Bombs

Day 6. Ricotta Cloud Pancakes - Parmesan Brussels Sprouts Salad - Asparagus Fries - Chicken Curry with Masala Keto Peanut Butter Chocolate Bars

Day 7. Keto Cinnamon Coffee - Shrimp and Avocado Lettuce Cups - Kale Chips - Chicken Quesadilla - Salted Toffee Nut Cups

Day 8. Keto Waffles and Blueberries - Keto Quesadillas - Guacamole - Slow Cooker Barbecue Ribs - Crisp Meringue Cookies

Day 9. Baked Avocado Eggs - No-Bread Italian Subs - Zucchini Noodles - Barbacoa Beef Roast - Instant Pot Matcha Cheesecake

Day 10. Mushroom Omelet - Turkey Meatballs - Cauliflower Soufflé - Beef & Broccoli Roast - Matcha Skillet Soufflé

Day 11. Keto Waffles and Blueberries - Cauliflower Leek Soup - Fried Green Beans Rosemary - Portobello Pizza Keto and Dairy-Free Vanilla Custard

Day 12. Baked Avocado Eggs - Blueberry Cottage Cheese Parfaits - Cheesy Cauliflower Croquettes - Turkey Mozzarella Burgers - Keto Triple Chocolate Mug Cake

Day 13. Baked Avocado Eggs - Blueberry Cottage Cheese Parfaits - Cheesy Cauliflower Croquettes - Turkey Mozzarella Burgers - Keto Triple Chocolate Mug Cake

Day 14. Almond Coconut Egg Wraps - Low-Carb Broccoli Leek Soup - Spinach in Cheese Envelopes - Grilled Chicken Salad with Oranges - Crisp Meringue Cookies

Day 15. Creamy Basil Baked Sausage - Low-Carb Chicken Taco Soup - Cheesy Mushroom Slices - Classic Chicken Salad - Instant Pot Matcha Cheesecake

DAY --> BREAKFAST --> LUNCH --> SNAK --> DINNER --> DESSERT

Day 16. Creamy Basil Baked Sausage - Low-Carb Chicken Taco Soup - Cheesy Mushroom Slices - Classic Chicken Salad - Instant Pot Matcha Cheesecake

Day 17. Baked Avocado Eggs - Low-Carb Seafood Soup with Mayo - Zucchini Noodles - Baked Cauliflower - Keto Cheesecake Stuffed Brownies

Day 18. Mushroom Omelet - Keto Tortilla Chips - Cauliflower Soufflé - Salmon Keto Cutlets - Crisp Meringue Cookies

Day 19. Coconut Keto Porridge - Chicken Zucchini Alfredo - Asparagus Fries - Italian Keto Casserole - Instant Pot Matcha Cheesecake

Day 20. Cheesy Bacon & Egg Cups - Low Carbs Chicken Cheese - Fried Green Beans Rosemary - Risotto with Mushrooms - Matcha Skillet Soufflé

Day 21. Ricotta Cloud Pancakes - Parmesan Brussels Sprouts Salad - Kale Chips - Low Carb Green Bean Casserole - Keto and Dairy-Free Vanilla Custard

Day 22. Keto Cinnamon Coffee - Caprese Zoodles - Guacamole - Grilled Chicken Salad with Oranges - Keto Triple Chocolate Mug Cake

Day 23. Almond Coconut Egg Wraps - chicken Tacos - Spinach in Cheese Envelopes - Buttery Garlic Chicken - Keto Cheesecake Stuffed Brownies

Day 24. Cream cheese eggs - No-Bread Italian Subs - Cheesy Mushroom Slices - Classic Chicken Salad - Matcha Skillet Soufflé

Day 25. Creamy Basil Baked Sausage - Turkey Meatballs - fried Green Beans Rosemary - Creamy Slow Cooker Chicken - Keto and Dairy-Free Vanilla Custard

Day 26. Coconut Keto Porridge - Blueberry Cottage Cheese Parfaits - Zucchini Noodles - Chicken Fillet with Brussel Sprouts - Keto Triple Chocolate Mug Cake

Day 27. Ricotta Cloud Pancakes - Cheesy Broccoli Quiche - Cauliflower Soufflé - Portobello Pizza - Keto and Dairy-Free Vanilla Custard

Day 28. Cheesy Bacon & Egg Cups - Low-Carb Broccoli Leek Soup - Cheesy Mushroom Slices - Turkey Mozzarella Burgers - Keto Raspberry Ice Cream

Day 29. Mushroom Omelet - Keto Chicken & Veggies Soup - Asparagus Fries - Grilled Chicken Salad with Oranges - Instant Pot Matcha Cheesecake

Day 30. Keto Cinnamon Coffee - Keto Tortilla Chips - Cheesy Mushroom Slices - Beef & Broccoli Roast - Keto Triple Chocolate Mug Cake

Conclusion

Your dedication to improve your health and lose weight is phenomenal since you have been able to reach the end of this guidebook. While it is hard to lose weight, if you can maintain the guidelines you have learned in this guidebook and stay motivated, your life will change in ways that you cannot imagine. You are on the right path in getting both mental and physical health. Even though adjusting to eating a healthy diet after being accustomed to eating a lot of convenience foods is a challenge; you will feel the difference in energy levels that you will experience. You will look good and be safe from many of the common nutrition-related diseases and conditions, and besides of all that, your quality of life will improve significantly.

We are all different; thus, you should take time to really understand what a weight loss program involves and try out the program gradually. If you nosedive into a weight loss program is not advisable since it may not be for you. No regiment works perfectly for everyone; thus, you should select a plan and modify it in a way that suits you. There are many weight loss programs with mind-blowing results, but they may be too hard to follow or just unsafe to practice.

Your workout intensity, the duration, and your resting period are all factors that should be considered. It works best when it is a constant in your daily activities, and as it is not a permanent change of your physical and psychological condition.

To get the maximum weight loss experience, you should listen to your body. It means that you should pay attention to how it responds to your diet and fasting regiment because the body system determines the time for you to eat, time for you to exercise and even how many calories you take in. Thus you will be in full control of your weight loss once you are in control of your diet and fasting program.

You should know that even though the ketogenic diet is about carbohydrate restriction, it doesn't excessively restrict them. You should make sure you eat enough. If you avoid food with calories too much, you will be moody, and it can even stop your weight loss process. You should also vary your food choices so that you make sure that you are getting the nutrients that your body needs to maintain a good healthy lifestyle.

Getting all the nutrients that you require from a ketogenic diet is possible. Unfortunately for some, this is not possible. If you do not feel okay, you should go and see a doctor to determine if you have any nutritional deficiencies. He/she will be able to recommend supplements for you from that information.

For health reasons, weight loss should be a slow process. Losing 2 pounds a day is okay, but anything more than that is too much. Engage in your day-to-day occupations while fasting as this is a time-flying route. Good luck with your keto diet journey!

THANK YOU

Finally, if you enjoyed this book, then I'd like to ask you for a favor, would you be kind enough to leave a review for this book on Amazon? It'd be greatly appreciated!

It would be crucial to help me with this project that I care about a lot. I believe that regardless of the book and the mission that matters. Everybody deserves a healthier and more just life. Maybe people are not aware of it.

Maybe we can help.

With Love,

Jillian Collins

GRAB YOUR 7 SPECIAL BONUS HERE!

https://7fastbonuses-KetoDiet50.gr8.com/

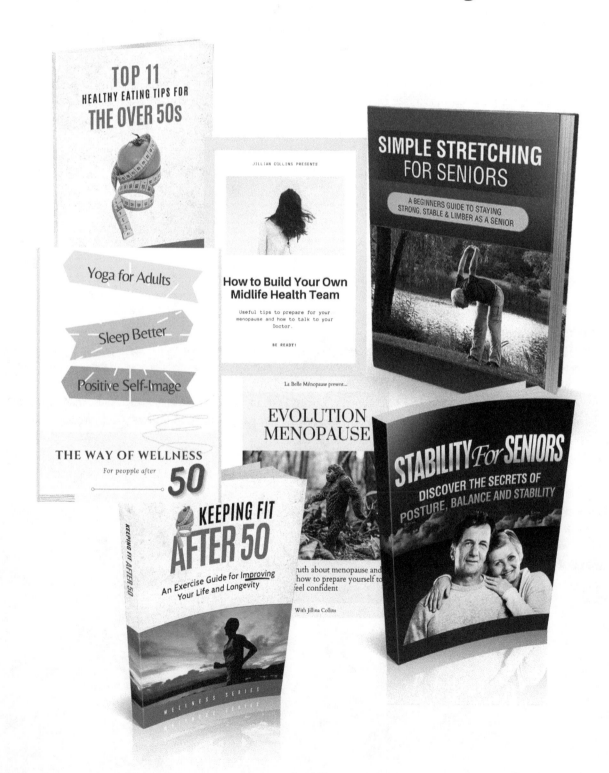

CPSIA information can be obtained
at www.ICGtesting.com
Printed in the USA
BVHW061816130421
604817BV00008B/425

9 781801 207485